Testosterone

A Simple and Practical Guide to Get You Back in the Game

(How to Boost Your Testosterone Levels in Different Ways Naturally)

Daniel Goodwin

Published By **Jackson Denver**

Daniel Goodwin

Testosterone: A Simple and Practical Guide to Get You Back in the Game (How to Boost Your Testosterone Levels in Different Ways Naturally)

ISBN 978-1-998927-44-9

Legal & Disclaimer

Table Of Contents

Chapter 1: Natural Methods to Boost Testosterone

Increasing natural testosterone stages within the body is regular and frequently powerful possibility to testosterone gels and injections, that could reason unwanted thing consequences.

This ebook is for men who're looking to improve their nicely-being, virility and strength thru growing testosterone stages in the frame via natural mechanisms. We will fine speak hooked up techniques and facts received from peer-reviewed medical journals and health technological expertise-orientated websites. In this way, best herbal strategies proven to boost testosterone regular with scientific proof is referred to. This ebook is an opportunity for all guys to enhance testosterone degrees in a herbal and regular manner.

The testosterone lab take a look at - described

A serum testosterone check is the best manner to determine the amount of testosterone hormone in our bloodstream. In this check, a blood sample is accumulated among 7 am to ten am – intervals wherein testosterone stages are maximum[11]. Because testosterone ranges in the blood modifications in the path of the day, numerous tests are needed in advance than the clinical doctor can give up a deficiency exists. It isn't uncommon for scientific docs to moreover order additional assessments to determine the fitness reputation of various endocrine organs as nicely.

A testosterone lab check is the high-quality way to diploma testosterone stages properly and because it have to be, and it cannot be measured over the internet or via using clearly answering quizzes or questionnaires.

The stop end result of testosterone check is regularly depicted inside the following:

•Total testosterone – the complete quantity of testosterone within the complete body, which includes those that are certain within the protein known as SHBG (intercourse hormone-binding globulin).

•Free testosterone – the quantity of testosterone not sure to SHBG, for this reason the term 'free' due to the fact it is more to be had to the frame.

The following are established regular degrees of testosterone in men over 19 years of age[12]:

•Total testosterone   240-950 ng/dL

•Free testosterone   20-29 years: 83-257 ng/dL

      30-39 years: seventy two-235 ng/dL

      40-forty nine years: 61-213 ng/dL

      50-fifty nine years: 50-one hundred ninety ng/dL

      60-69 years: 40-168 ng/dL

Now that we've included some of the facts about the values measured in serum testosterone test, it's also crucial to be familiar with medical conditions that have an impact on testosterone stages and male virility.

Causes for Low Testosterone

There are a few conditions that specify why guys suffer from low testosterone. This is the motive why men who are suspecting as such, need to first go to a scientific health practitioner for a thorough scientific evaluation.

Here are sure medical situations that would cause depressed testosterone tiers and virility:

Old age

Testosterone decline takes area on numerous factors. One of the most commonplace is because of developing old. It is natural for men to revel in a decline in testosterone stages as they age. Testosterone stages naturally drop in guys (and girls) as we age in keeping with a observe posted in The Journal of Urology[13]. According to the Reviews in Urology, it is set up that guys enjoy a 1% decline in testosterone tiers each yr by the time they acquire 30 years of age[14]. How this takes place to developing old person men remains now not but understood. Because of this, older guys have a tendency to have lower testosterone degrees compared to their extra younger contrary numbers.

But a cutting-edge day have a observe published with the aid of the Endocrine Society states that testosterone decline is extra associated with presence of terrible behaviors (this will be elaborated later) so consequently growing old doesn't continually advocate cut price in testosterone or virility[15]. So it is viable to preserve immoderate testosterone levels, irrespective of ones age.

Diabetes

Men with kind-2 diabetes will be predisposed to have low testosterone tiers in assessment to their more healthful counterparts. In a look at published in magazine Diabetes Care, 50% of obese diabetic men have lower-than-normal degrees of unfastened testosterone[16]. Low testosterone-person men moreover have a tendency to have adverse metabolic profile like impaired glucose tolerance and excessive insulin resistance (signs and symptoms of pre-diabetes)[17]. Low testosterone tiers play a role in development of insulin resistance that outcomes to diabetes[18]. Still, weight reduction and workout can help testosterone-poor diabetic men enhance their testosterone degrees and virility[19].

Obesity

Men who're overweight also face chance of having low testosterone stages[20]. A very present day day test confirmed that obese pubertal and put up-pubertal person adult males have testosterone levels that are forty-50% lower in evaluation to grownup men with more wholesome weight[21], which best confirm findings from earlier research. Like in diabetes, low testosterone is also a predictor to weight troubles in guys[22].

Cancer treatment

For men present manner or have handed through maximum cancers remedy, they will enjoy reduced testosterone levels. This is usually an negative impact of many chemotherapeutic drug treatments[23]. Some maximum cancers treatments, like prostate surgical procedure, belly surgical remedy and lymph node elimination, or maybe ensuing in sexual dysfunction because of nerves and blood vessels that innervate the penis being removed[24].

Hypertension

Persistent immoderate blood strain additionally lowers testosterone and destroys male virility. Hypertension on the issue of immoderate cholesterol levels and weight issues are predictive factors for low testosterone, in step with a take a look at published in International Journal of

Impotence Research[25]. In addition, low testosterone is placed to be related hypertension and weird increase of the left aspect of the coronary heart constant with a observe in European Journal of Endocrinology[26]. Hypertension additionally may be the cause why many men have hassle very last hard for prolonged durations of time (erectile sickness), in step with a take a look at within the magazine Hypertension[27]. This locating is supported via way of a have a observe wherein it's miles decided that guys with excessive blood pressure engage in 25% an entire lot lots much less sexual interest in step with month in contrast to greater healthy guys[28].

History of beyond damage to the testicles, mumps orchitis, hemochromatosis, and chemotherapy also can purpose reduction of testosterone ranges[29]. Furthermore, some drug treatments like statins, antidepressants, antihypertensives and antiepileptic medicinal capsules are recognized to lower testosterone in guys[30][31]. Many of these medical situations are not unusual in guys, that is every different vital reason a medical checkup want to be completed in the first vicinity.

Improving testosterone absolutely can assist men who are stricken by the above-stated medical conditions. Testosterone has many capabilities other than its famous use as muscle builder and virility the usage of pressure. Testosterone promotes resilience of bones and improves mentally alertness and ordinary health.

Despite rumors, testosterone is actually tested to lessen cardiovascular disease in aged men. Normal testosterone ranges moreover have protective effect in competition to neurodegenerative conditions which encompass Alzheimer's sickness and dementia[32]. These are some of the few unique reasons why guys want to make certain they will be producing accurate sufficient testosterone within the route in their complete lifestyles.

Chapter 2: Testosterone Boosting Foods

It is feasible to seriously adjust our testosterone diploma through way of in reality changing the ingredients we consume. Many ingredients have been tested to dramatically reduce testosterone degrees at the same time as distinct ingredients had been verified to dramatically growth testosterone. Any guy looking to enhance his testosterone levels must glaringly consume more testosterone-boosting factors and decreasing the consumption of testosterone destroying additives.

We will now start with the useful resource of mentioning the various food that might beautify testosterone production for men.

Testosterone-boosting food

Some meals can beautify testosterone truely due to the fact they supply critical nutrients wanted thru the body which may be used within the production of testosterone. Keep in mind that the primary producer of testosterone in the body, the testes, are constantly at art work producing sperm cells and sex hormones and consequently need a everyday supply of those vitamins. Many men are poor in the ones important vitamins, resulting in lower testosterone stages and virility. In fact, vitamin and mineral deficiencies are a leading purpose of low testosterone and terrible virility in guys.

Often touted as "aphrodisiacs", some of the ones components provide the frame with these crucial key nutrients ensuing in better natural manufacturing of testosterone and expanded sexual normal performance in guys, as supported thru those research:

Oysters

Oysters are extended touted during information as effective aphrodisiacs[33][34]. What data has been telling us about the sexual powers of oysters may be actual, in keeping with medical studies. Oysters are high in zinc, and are the richest meals supply of this mineral[35].

Zinc could be very vital for the reproductive fitness in guys, or even a slight deficiency of this mineral has an impact on testosterone tiers. In a study posted within the mag Nutrition, it is located that restriction of zinc brought about testosterone ranges to drop in as little as 20 weeks, and further supplementation of the mineral helped opposite it[36]. Another take a look at posted in American Journal of Hematology showed that zinc can increase serum testosterone ranges in men affected by sickle-mobile anemia[37]. Even amongst grownup guys with infertility troubles, greater zinc supplementation furthermore helped improve testosterone degrees and sperm counts drastically[38]. Exhaustive bodily activity also can decrease blood testosterone, but this has been proven to be reversed by using using way of zinc supplementation[39].

To boom testosterone degrees, consume one serving of oysters (one serving is 3 ounces) consistent with day. This has about seventy 4 mg of zinc in it. Cooking oysters in liquid can also reason the zinc to leach out, so it's miles top notch to devour them raw or baked.

Beef

Steaks of pork are a well-known fare for men and research indicates men have to eat greater of it to in reality boom testosterone tiers. Lean cuts of pork are 2d simplest to oysters with regards to zinc content material material[40]. In addition, beef cuts are also excessive in selenium (more on this mineral later) which helps beautify sperm health for better fertility[41].

Eating pork is one of the most effective strategies to uplift zinc tiers in the body. Cook beef with out added fats, and reduce software program software of salt. To additionally avoid the leaching of vital vitamins, it is incredible to prepare dinner dinner tender cuts of red meat with out liquid.

Lean meat

We often pay attention from bodybuilders that lean protein can help enhance muscle development. Many health net websites suggests that red meat improves testosterone. According to a chunk of writing featured in Forbes, steaks ranked top amongst topics considered 'manly'[42]. This is based completely totally on a observe posted in Journal of Consumer Research, wherein it have become decided that respondents implied that meat eaters are greater masculine than non-meat eaters[43]. Lean meat is high in protein and there are gift research which show that it is able to have a effective impact on testosterone ranges.

A hormone called SHBG (sex hormone-binding globulin) is inversely associated with protein intake because of this that if a food plan is low in protein then SHBG levels rises, in line with a research have a examine concerning 1,552 men[44]. SHBG binds to the testosterone inside the bloodstream, and is the cause why testosterone assessments effects display sure testosterone (T effective in SHBG) and 'free' testosterone (unbound T). High degrees of SHBG propose that extra testosterone is caught inside the bloodstream in area of going to aim tissues like muscle agencies and gonads, that would result in symptoms of low testosterone even though tiers are nicely sufficient or everyday[45]. This shows that eating extra protein from lean meat allows decrease SHBG so more testosterone will become available to the body.

Protein sources need to be low in fat, due to the reality stepped forward lipid ranges and excessive body weight can show terrible to testosterone. A cut of beef roasted, is a high-quality example of lean meat. Other appropriate lean protein-wealthy fare examples are beef and chicken (with out pores and skin and seen fat) and recreation meats like venison.

Brazil nuts

Brazil nuts are excessive in selenium. In animal research, selenium proved to help defend the body from reproductive toxicities delivered approximately thru pesticides, ethanol and nicotine in male rabbits and rats[46][47][48]. In a examine posted in Journal of Andrology, selenium helped improve sperm motility in wholesome men[49]. Selenium additionally improved semen extraordinary developments, consistent with a check in The Journal of Urology[50]. Selenium is likewise idea to enhance testosterone production which may also deliver an reason behind why it's far beneficial for men with fertility problems, in line with a take a look at in Nigeria[51].

Six to 8 quantities of Brazil nuts make one serving, which has 544 micrograms of selenium. Only a few portions want to be eaten every special day to assist enhance low testosterone ranges.

Chapter 3: Swordfish, salmon and cod liver oil

Fish oil dietary dietary supplements are one of the maximum popular supplements inside the market. Certain fish oils, substantially swordfish, salmon and cod liver oil can decorate testosterone in numerous strategies. These fish oils are immoderate in vitamins D[52], which in line with specialists can decorate testosterone in men.

Despite being called a 'sunshine weight-reduction plan', it's far very difficult for men to get enough vitamins D from sunlight hours if dwelling at better latitudes, generally generally tend to cowl while underneath the solar, use sunscreens frequently, have darker skin tone or overweight[53]. Vitamin D is handiest to be had in tiny quantities in tuna, fortified orange juice, cereals and milk. However, the richest source of nutrients D in our diet comes from cod liver oil[54].

There are severa human research showing that nutrition D has impact concerning testosterone degrees within the frame, consistent with the test within the magazine Reproduction[55]. Men who have regular weight loss plan D ranges normally will be predisposed to have higher stages of serum testosterone too[56].

Cod liver is likewise an notable source of healthful fats in the weight loss program, and exact sufficient intake of fats is needed for correct production of testosterone in the testicles, that is supported by the usage of manner of numerous studies in step with a piece of writing featured within the magazine Nutrients[57]. In addition, cod liver is also a wealthy supply of nutrition A. In a have a study featured in Clinical Endocrinology, eating regimen A with iron is shown to be as powerful as hormonal remedy to result in boom and puberty in male kids with pubertal put off (take note that testosterone induces puberty)[58].

Cod liver oil is likewise strongly anti inflammatory, this means that that that that it reduces amounts of contamination-inflicting markers within the blood[59]. Studies display that there is an association amongst infection and low testosterone tiers[60][61].

Fish oils are regularly available in dietary supplements. Baking or broiling clean cod, salmon and swordfish is also a recommended way to eat fish oils. You need to have at the least 500 IU of vitamins D consistent with day, and for most appropriate testosterone tiers, you may need at the least six hundred IU a day. As a guide, one serving (three oz) of swordfish and salmon has 566 mcg and 447 mcg of diet regime D, respectively, whilst 7 mL of (half tablespoon) of liver cod oil has 680 IU.

Garlic

Garlic is a prized spice and remedy due to the fact the sunrise of statistics. Garlic is known and used in almost all Eurasian cultures – historical Egypt, Greece and Rome, India, China and Korea. All of those historic cultures diagnosed the medicinal houses of garlic and prescribed it for severa ailments[62]. Modern research suggests that garlic is beneficial for high blood pressure, superior blood glucose and additionally for reinforcing testosterone levels.

Recent research moreover show that garlic is useful to testosterone tiers, in particular while consumed in a immoderate-protein weight loss program[63]. Another examine confirmed that dehydrated garlic powder and uncooked garlic juice enables recover testicular characteristic and spermatogenesis, which means this spice has been tested to be effective at boosting herbal testosterone production[64]. Testosterone can also spark off high blood strain[65], however because of the truth garlic can lessen blood stress, it's far recommended to be included in normal weight-reduction plan for men.

Based on severa studies, garlic is splendid consumed uncooked. An remarkable manner to devour raw garlic is via which includes it in salads. Make a extraordinarily spiced salad by means of using way of mixing chopped garlic with tomatoes, onion and ginger and basil and a few vegetable oil. Instead of mayo, combo pressed garlic with egg yolk and mix until easy. To help lessen the ugly odor (garlic breath) which comes from eating raw garlic, keep in mind eating it with fats-containing liquid like olive oil, milk or cream.

Pomegranate

Historically, pomegranate is related to fertility and fruitfulness (in human reproduction, I wager)[66]. Pomegranate arils are wealthy in vitamins, minerals and fiber plus it incorporates loads of antioxidants[67][68]. This wholesome and great fruit is likewise recounted to improve testosterone consistent with modern day studies.

According to analyze in rats, pomegranates helped enhance antioxidant stage, male reproductive characteristic and testosterone degrees[69]. In a totally extremely-present day have a test posted inside the mag Endocrine Abstracts, volunteer human subjects given pomegranate juice for two weeks exhibited raised salivary testosterone tiers, and it furthermore advanced mood, blood stress and anxiety tiers[70].

Not all pomegranate juices offered are identical because of the reality a number of them are loaded with food coloring and sugar. It is exceptional to apply sparkling pomegranates to make pomegranate juice. To make sparkling pomegranate juice, lessen the whole fruit in half of, make numerous cuts at the rind, flip the halves over a bowl and smack with a spoon to separate the arils from the inedible pulp. The complete approach want to most effective take 10-20 seconds consistent with half of of pomegranate and it's far an exceptionally powerful approach of putting apart the inedible pulp from the arils at the same time as no longer having to play around and select out it out by the usage of using hand. Add pomegranate arils to candy desserts and smoothies, or encompass them in vegetable salads.

Chapter 4: Cruciferous greens

There is considerable proof that cruciferous veggies like cabbage, broccoli, Brussels sprouts, kale and bok choy help manual testosterone degrees[71]. Cruciferous greens are already identified as mainly nutritious veggies due to their blessings to health[72]. Cruciferous greens incorporate indole-3-carbinol, which have already got numerous documented beneficial homes within the frame[73].

In a have a study published within the Journal of the National Cancer Institute, it discovered that human topics given indole-3-carbinol confirmed multiplied secretion of estrogen metabolites (by-product materials left after estrogen modified into used inside the body). Several studies additionally confirmed the anti-estrogenic houses of indole-3-carbinol, consistent with The Journal of Nutrition[74]. Estrogen is the number one intercourse characteristic hormone in ladies and furthermore placed in men, and for the length of getting older, the quantity of estrogen will increase in guys at the fee of testosterone ranges[75]. Since indole-three-carbinol improves excretion of estrogen via-merchandise, it helps lessen estrogen and enhance testosterone tiers, presenting a herbal remedy for hormonal balancing.

For elevated testosterone production, bear in mind eating at least servings of cruciferous greens an afternoon. Get the entire dietary advantages of cruciferous greens via eating them raw or lightly steamed. Broccoli, kale and Brussels sprouts may be very well eaten raw, and they lend well flavor and crunch to salads, casseroles or maybe sandwiches. Do now not overcook cruciferous vegetables because it leaches nutrients in steam and the water it's far cooked in, plus they scent unappetizing. Always pick cruciferous veggies which can be deeply colored; having red, dark inexperienced or bluish hue due to the reality as they'll likely consist of a better quantity of useful vitamins.

Honey

Honey is one of the richest resources of boron[76]. Boron is a hint mineral in recent times located to enhance testosterone tiers in the body. There also are studies showing that honey can decorate nitric acid stages within the bloodstream. In the frame, nitric acid is chargeable for dilating blood vessels[77]. This dilating movement performs an crucial characteristic in erections of the penis; the dilation of the arteries inside the penis permits blood to gather and engorge the penis to reason an erection[78]. Sildenafil citrate, better called Viagra, furthermore works this manner and became at the beginning permitted as a hypertensive drug because it dilates the blood vessels, however it also advanced erection in men that paved for its in addition use as a drug for erectile sickness[79].

In an test on women, supplementation of boron furthermore extended serum testosterone degrees in ladies[80]. Another have a have a look at posted in The British Journal of Nutrition installed that improved boron consumption in weight loss program improves testosterone in girls volunteers[81]. In a test achieved in Dubai, intake of honey raised saliva, urine and blood nitric oxide tiers internal three hours after ingestion[82]. A have a study posted in 2011 confirmed that volunteers who took boron dietary supplements exhibited decreased intercourse-hormone binding globulin (SHBG, the most effective that holds testosterone in bloodstream) and inflammatory materials on the same time as at the equal time elevated hormone production together with testosterone[83].

Therefore, men can use this candy and sticky stuff to enhance testosterone ranges further to decorate ordinary performance during intercourse. Honey is a high-quality palate purifier. It is likewise viable to apply honey in location of sugar on every occasion viable. For a healthy snack, honey can be drizzled on stop cease result and berries. The pleasant element is there's no expiry date on honey - it has a shelf lifestyles greater than our lifetime.

Even honey located in the historical Egyptian tomb had now not spoiled - even after 2,000 years.

Whole eggs

Many health-orientated net net sites factor out eggs as someone's excellent buddy for testosterone tiers. There is not any research straight away linking consumption of eggs to improvement of testosterone degrees. However, deeper assessment of the dietary profile of hen eggs suggests that it does help testosterone tiers within the frame.

Eggs are a deliver of weight-reduction plan D and it is placed particularly inside the yolk[84]. As said in advance, extra supplementation of weight loss program D can help growth testosterone stages[85][86]. Eggs moreover have big amount of calcium, even in case you do not devour the shell[87]. Eggs furthermore have simply the proper serving of fat and calcium, which is likewise supportive for testosterone ranges[88][89].

Improve testosterone by using the use of way of consuming one egg a day, ideally with out more fat at the identical time as cooking. Have a boiled egg for breakfast or for a snack. It is also feasible to toss slices of boiled egg with cruciferous greens as a virility-improving snack. For guys concerned about the more energy, its essential those ingredients are ate up alongside an workout regiment - moreover mentioned inner this ebook (which is ideal for compounding boosting natural testosterone results of food and exercise).

Yogurt

There is big proof which shows that yogurt can assist beautify testosterone degrees. Consuming yogurt is already considered healthy due to the reality historical instances[90]. In an animal look at, mice that have been given yogurt had big testicles and inseminated girl mice faster and more regularly in assessment to mice given a junk-food based totally food regimen[91]. Yogurt furthermore has huge quantities of protein, it virtually is greater than the equal quantity of whole milk. Protein is connected to enhancements in testosterone regular with a few studies[92][93].

As for the type of yogurt, it's miles wonderful to consume low-fat and coffee-sugar yogurt for the easy cause it does no longer encompass big portions of sugar and fats. Avoid flavored yogurt or manufacturers with blended 'culmination' because of the reality they're likely sweetened with immoderate-fructose corn syrup; don't forget it's miles important to keep frame weight in check for max testosterone production. Use yogurt in dips, or definitely add chopped glowing cease end result and consume as a deal with. For those men attempting to find to sweeten their yogurt, remember honey as an possibility sweetener to compound the testosterone boosting effects of those two excellent meals assets.

Oats

Oats can be beneficial for testosterone. Oat flakes are immoderate in L-arginine[94]. A eating regimen excessive in l-arginine is related to superior sexual function in men, in keeping with many studies[95]. L-arginine within the frame is transformed into nitric oxide (which changed into cited earlier as essential thing in preserving sturdy erections[96]). In a take a look at posted within the Journal of Endocrinology, dietary arginine is critical in the manufacturing of testosterone in the frame[97].

Oats are filling and may be a part of a healthy breakfast or snack object. Prepare oats with out added sugar as lots as feasible. Instead, recall eating oats with different testosterone-boosting meals which includes honey, nuts and pomegranates.

Chapter 5: Chickpeas

Chickpeas have additionally shown to decorate testosterone and it's miles believed that is due to the reality they may be rich in zinc, a mineral that plays an crucial role in hormone production and spermatogenesis. Zinc is likewise to be had in more commonplace substances like complete grains, legumes and beans[98]. However, the ones meals incorporate immoderate amounts of the antinutrient phytic acid which absolutely prevents minerals like zinc from being absorbed within the body[99]. Among food belongings, chickpeas have the lowest amount of phytic acid, so it's far a primary source of zinc.

Men with low testosterone generally have a tendency to have poor tiers of zinc inside the body[100]. Men with gonadal deficiency because of uremia superior their testosterone stages and sexual ordinary typical overall performance with the aid of manner of supplementation of zinc[101]. Furthermore, it's miles determined that the reproductive feature and serum testosterone ranges in guys are touchy to zinc degree fluctuations[102]. Therefore, it's miles crucial for all men to insure they have got suitable enough degrees of zinc - a common hassle placed inside the path of this ebook.

Soaking chickpeas in water in advance than cooking can power down phytic acid degree as a way to increase bioavailability of zinc within the body. Chickpeas can be boiled until easy, then mashed and mixed with olive oil, lemon and sesame seed paste, juice, salt and garlic to make tasty hummus.

Irradiated mushrooms

There is proof that eating more irradiated mushrooms can beautify testosterone levels. These are mushrooms which can be subjected to ultraviolet B rays. Irradiated mushrooms aren't subjected to dangerous ionizing radiation, so they will be flawlessly secure to consume. Ordinary mushrooms incorporate small portions of vitamins D. But exposing mushrooms to pulses of ultraviolet-B radiation will growth their nutrients D content material by way of using as plenty as 824%. There is proof that vitamins D enables hold and beautify testosterone levels in the frame. A have a study posted in the magazine Clinical Endocrinology showed that guys with adequate tiers of nutrition D have better testosterone stages[103]. Another current have a examine shows that, in desire to a placebo, supplementation of weight loss plan D helped growth testosterone tiers in men with diabetes[104].

For those guys who live a long way from the equator, use sunscreen or have darkish pores and pores and skin, it's far quite viable they may be affected by eating regimen D deficiency. Only few animal sources have ok amounts of eating regimen D. Fortunately, almost all varieties of mushrooms, inclusive of desk mushrooms, white mushrooms, oyster and shitake mushrooms, may be irradiated[105] and provide an wonderful opportunity deliver of diet D.

Testosterone stages can be elevated by using manner of manner of consuming a serving of irradiated mushrooms each day. Vitamin D is a fat-soluble nutrients, so it's miles brilliant to put together mushrooms via together with some fat or oil. The mushrooms may be sliced and sautéed with veggies and thin slices of meat with little oil. Mushrooms additionally can be brought to soups, burgers, sandwiches and roasts.

Avocado

This yummy and healthful oil-rich fruit has fitness homes that could assist beautify testosterone and likely save a person's life and manhood. Avocado incorporates healthy fats that can enhance your ldl ldl cholesterol profile via developing HDL (excessive-density lipoprotein, the outstanding ldl ldl cholesterol) and decreasing LDL (low-density lipoprotein, the artery-blocking ldl cholesterol). Good ldl ldl cholesterol profile is vital because of the truth steady with a population-based totally test published in

Arteriosclerosis, Thrombosis and Vascular Biology, ok degrees of HDL is associated with better ordinary testosterone in men[106]. It is crucial to never underestimate the impact of high blood stress - due to the fact it could negatively have an impact on the blood drift to the penis, consistent with a have a have a look at posted in Journal of Urology[107]. Furthermore erectile disease is extra regularly taking place in guys with high blood pressure, consistent with contemporary-day research in Egyptian and Qatari guys[108][109]. Thus, those studies show that avocados can be very beneficial for maintaining up testosterone ranges, reduce chances of coronary heart sicknesses (existence saving traits) and reduce risk of laid low with erectile disorder.

Avocado is also a delectable and wholesome opportunity for fats in common dishes. Consume avocado through using it in place of butter in sandwiches. One encouraged way to devour avocado is to puree it, then use in vicinity of mayonnaise in sandwiches, salads and bloodless cuts. Make delicious and healthful guacamole through way of using mixing avocado with chopped onions, tomatoes, garlic, lime and chili and a few salt.

Grapes

Grapes additionally can be correct for max testosterone manufacturing. We refer proper proper right here to grapes that are fed on complete, for instance desk grapes. The skins of grapes incorporate resveratrol, a phenol which have numerous effects at the frame. Animal research display that resveratrol will growth testosterone[110][111]. In a take a look at in rats posted in The Journal of Nutrition, rats fed with resveratrol showed advanced sperm production and higher testosterone stages in comparison to govern rats[112].

This indicates intake of grapes might also additionally have incredible effects on your testosterone and sperm extremely good. Eat the ones grapes glowing or frozen. It is also feasible to feature grapes to oats and yogurt to sweeten breakfast dishes, as properly makes an first rate lunch time snack and healthful dinner dessert food.

Butter from grass-fed cows

The additives in butter from grass-fed cows may be beneficial to testosterone. Butter from grass-fed cows is evidently herbal and includes excessive levels of carotenoids[113]. Compared to butter from feedlot livestock, butter from grass-fed cows is excessive in omega-three fatty acids[114]. A weight-reduction plan exact sufficient in omega-3 fatty acids permits manage immoderate ldl ldl ldl cholesterol, excessive blood pressure and decrease chance of atherosclerosis[115][116] – elements which have all been implicated in lowering testosterone degrees.

Chapter 6: Organic end result and vegetables

We will take take a look at right right here of the importance of eating natural end result and greens. It is essential to understand that pesticides utilized in agriculture pose risk to our fitness, and studies display that it moreover lowers testosterone and sperm first rate in guys. Carbosulfan, a extensively used pesticide, go away residues in meals and is decided to purpose sperm malformations and reduce testosterone in rabbits[118][119]. Pesticides in agriculture are located to reason infertility and occasional testosterone tiers in human beings[120][121]. The significance of heading off the consumption of these insecticides generally located on our fruit and greens cannot be emphasised sufficient!

Men excessive approximately enhancing natural testosterone production need to subsist on organic fruits and greens. They may cost a little barely greater, however the benefits obtained are large. It is viable to save extra with the beneficial resource of buying natural meals locally and at farmer's markets. Buying natural meals is also much less complex and lots less highly-priced if shopping for merchandise which can be in season.

All the elements we mentioned proper proper here will assist you recognize how ingesting proper lets in to sincerely beautify testosterone tiers. As stated in advance, it is crucial to consume greater testosterone-boosting elements in region of an awful lot a lot less nutritious and completely avoid the testosterone destroying food (subsequent phase).

It is normally vital to examine the endorsed servings and be vigilant about calorie counts due to the reality too much body weight is also a cause of low testosterone. Therefore, it is crucial to be careful what is eaten and to in no way over indulge, particularly on regarded testosterone destroying meals. Men who're overweight want to furthermore hold in mind a weight manipulate software because of the truth fat loss additionally permits to boost natural testosterone stages.

Testosterone Destroying Foods

Aside from consuming meals which have been validated to honestly growth testosterone tiers, it is also crucial to recognize that there are various elements that decrease testosterone ranges. Some components may also want to have the sort of terrible impact on testosterone levels that male virility is also notably effected in a bad manner. Many of the meals referred to right here are extensively eaten, which may moreover additionally provide an purpose behind why such plenty of fellows these days are laid low with low testosterone and virility problems. It is well well really worth noting that men with decrease-than-ordinary testosterone typically have a tendency to report low sex electricity and common bad penile erection[122].

Here are the food items that harm virility, which every person want to keep away from:

Beer and immoderate alcohol

Let's first begin with very famous and maximum common alcoholic drink for men - Beer. This is cited first due to the truth commercials frequently imbue beer with male virility. Beer commercials are pretty oriented towards men. However, studies says that beer isn't always brilliant for testosterone or virility in men.

Hops, the number one flavoring in beer, has a flavanone compound known as 8-prenylnaringenin (8-PN) which has immoderate estrogenic interest[123]. There also are exceptional estrogenic compounds in beer and hops[124]. Estrogen is the hormone that develops and facilitates woman inclinations in women and it counters the effects of testosterone. Beer can also furthermore encompass small quantities or only extracts of hops, so a bottle a day won't reason any large harm. But binge consuming booze ought to have a dramatic horrific effect on testosterone tiers, now not bringing up that it could moreover result in lousy performance within the mattress room[125]. Although beer can feature as a brilliant social lubricant and ice-breaker, too much is honestly detrimental to male not unusual typical overall performance and testosterone stages.

In addition, excessive alcohol intake ought to have degrading impact on testosterone, as evidenced by using using studies in rats[126][127]. A New England Journal of Medicine test furthermore showed that immoderate alcohol can also lower testosterone in people[128].

For guys tormented by low testosterone degrees, it's far going to be suitable to avoid ingesting beer all together. As a opportunity, one-of-a-type alcoholic drinks that do not include hops, which includes wine or vodka are options to bear in mind. For men looking for to boom testosterone, it's miles vital to decrease alcohol intake. For folks who do drink, take no more than one famous drink an afternoon (identical to 0.6 oz.. Or 14 grams of natural alcohol[129]) in keeping with day. More than that may considerably lessen blood testosterone ranges.

Soy products

Food merchandise made from soybeans are very well-known everywhere in the international, in particular in East Asia. Some examples of meals crafted from soy encompass soy sauce, tofu and edamame, textured vegetable protein (TVP, used as imitation meat) and plenty of extra. A lot of processed components include soybean-based genuinely products or soybean oil.

Despite its healthfulness, soy-primarily based definitely absolutely meals can be terrible on your testosterone. Soybeans are extensively rich in isoflavones, which have a robust estrogenic activity in the frame[130]. A have a examine published within the European Journal of Clinical Nutrition established how supplementation of soya flour reduced bloodstream testosterone in men[131].

Soybeans might not be able to without a doubt feminize guys, however it is able to have an effect on humans with already low testosterone degrees. Soybeans are healthy, but for men who've problems with low testosterone, any merchandise that incorporate soybeans or soybean oil need to be prevented. With so much processed meals and the huge amount of soy products used as a base factor in quite a few those materials, it's far crucial to scrutinize food labels carefully to appearance if it carries soybeans or has been processed in a facility that also techniques soybeans.

Beans and lentils

A every day bowl of lentils may offer an reason behind why a mans libido is slow. When talking about beans and lentils we are which incorporates the large definition of beans, collectively with pulses, legumes and peas. Let me say this right away – beans and lentils are healthy, however in line with many studies it is able to have a horrific effect on blood testosterone tiers[132][133].

In this regard, unique soluble fiber-wealthy substances like bran flakes, oats and complete grains can also prevent the growth of testosterone ranges. How this takes vicinity stays now not clean, but it's miles evident that high consumption of fiber can motive a awful impact on testosterone tiers. Inversely, a excessive-fat low-fiber eating regimen might also assist decorate testosterone levels in the blood, regular with an check posted in The American Journal of Clinical Nutrition[134]. Understandably this is in stark evaluation to the chant of the health food community over the last 50 years which states, "High Fiber, Low Fat" diets are tremendous for our fitness. If primitive guy's food plan is any indication of what our our bodies have superior to devour, then a diet plan rich in protein, fat and vegetables may additionally moreover possibly be the manner to transport. This concept reinforces the popularity of many diets which help this belief, along with the

Paleo diet, Primal, WAPF, Atkins and enormous form of others which can be gaining recognition.

It is essential to apprehend that we don't ought to live away truly from beans, lentils or whole grains – they're wholesome for you. Only ensure that smaller quantities and reduced frequency of servings of beans, lentils and entire grains are consumed in keeping with day. It is generally advocated to have no more than 1 serving of fiber a few instances an afternoon. For those craving fiber, attempt getting it from end result on the side of bananas and whole berries as an opportunity which may be food that have a much better nutrient density and are on the testosterone boosting problem of the equation.

Foods rich in salt

Let's be clear - an excessive amount of salt is awful for guys. This ought to no longer be facts to every person. However, most men are not aware that salty food even have a awful effect on testosterone degrees because it increases arterial blood pressure. It want to be delivered that elevated arterial blood pressure is likewise bad for mattress room overall performance, potentially reducing blood float to the penis.

There is compelling proof that excessive blood stress has a awful effect on serum testosterone. In rats, excessive blood strain is associated with decreased testosterone stages consistent with a have a study published in the magazine Endocrinology. Another have a take a look at posted in the Journal of Hypertension showed that excessive blood pressure can purpose testosterone tiers in guys to drop[135]. The effects of low testosterone is apparent in a test posted inside the American Journal of Hypertension, which confirmed that men with immoderate blood stress exhibited 25% discount in sexual interest similarly to twelve% cut price in serum testosterone.

Hypertension is exacerbated by using immoderate sodium intake and salty components are always immoderate in sodium. Therefore, high blood strain exacerbated through immoderate salt consumption can also moreover result in decreased testosterone levels for the ones men.

Salt intake have to be no more than a teaspoonful in keeping with day. It is smart to keep away from consuming an excessive amount of salt through staying a long way from processed meat and canned items, speedy-meals and clean drinks, and carnival food gadgets.

Chapter 7: Bottled water and meals wrapped in easy plastic

You also can have heard approximately BPA or bisphenol, right? BPA's are chemical substances widely used in the plastic agency, and it is determined in plastics collectively with water bottles, stick-wrap, resealable plastic meals containers and liners in canned tins[136]. BPAs make plastics easy, tough and impermeable, that are all nice packaging attributes inside the meals company.

However, near health, there are excellent research showing that BPA's can have an effect on fertility, and might probable have an effect on testosterone tiers inside the body. BPA is a regarded reproductive toxin that could reduce testosterone production and sperm counts in rats[137][138]. In each other take a look at in rats, BPA's reduced the amount of Leydig cells within the testes which produces testosterone[139]. Continuous control shows that BPA can virtually acquire in the frame, which could result in harming prolonged-term reproductive and endocrine functions[140].

Are you thinking that BPA can exceptional reduce testosterone in rats and no longer in men? There are already human studies displaying that BPA can lower testosterone stages in men[141][142][143]. BPA may additionally even cause sexual troubles in guys, it truly is associated with deficiency in testosterone[144].

All men need to be worried with defensive their testosterone tiers with the aid of reducing contact with products containing BPA. It is essential to avoid bottled water, and products which use smooth plastic programs for storing meals, chips or extraordinary food packaged in plastic or in plastic-blanketed packing containers. It is vital to carefully pick out BPA unfastened packing containers or as an opportunity glass bins for food and water garage and to avoid consuming bottled water as a good deal as feasible.

Foods excessive in saturated fat

Although many fatty meals are immoderate in ldl cholesterol, and ldl cholesterol is crucial for the manufacturing of testosterone, too much fatty ingredients can lessen common testosterone production and impair virility causing lower sperm counts in guys. Some famous fatty meals items embody bacon and processed meats, pasta-based totally dishes, cheese-based genuinely dishes, French-fried potatoes, ice cream and shakes, pot pies and fats-based totally salad dressings, and most American pizza dishes[145]. These meals gadgets make contributions to the very high-quality quantity of saturated fats inside the American healthy eating plan, and ingesting at the least such a devices (minimal of nineteen grams of popular fat regular with serving) can show horrific in your virility consistent with research.

In a have a test on Danish guys published in the magazine Human Reproduction, excessive consumption of fats within the healthy eating plan is correlated with cut price of sperm attention and counts[146]. This is supported with the aid of way of way of some different current have a check in American Journal of Clinical Nutrition showed that there is a dose-related association among intake of saturated fats and decrease sperm exceptional[147]. Reduction of intake of saturated fat is higher than disposing of them altogether within the weight loss plan, due to the reality there may be proof that low-fat weight-reduction plan can also reduce quantity of testosterone inside the body[148]. The critical remove from this research is nominal intake of fat within the weight-reduction plan is critical. Too low or too excessive is bad to our male fitness.

To regain virility and on the identical time provide the frame with the essential ldl cholesterol this is used for the manufacturing of testosterone, it's miles incredible vital to lessen the servings of fat-wealthy factors (no longer dispose of them altogether). Foods with loads of fat are ordinary observed in locations together with fast-meals joints, cinemas and carnivals. A lot of consolation food objects, like potato chips, sausages, shakes, and ice cream, pizza and pot pies also are rich in saturated fats. In alternate of lowering saturated fats-rich food, make certain to consume meals with unique styles of fats like omega-three that is more healthy for the body and does no longer lower testosterone or sperm counts.

Foods like soy and beans and lentils are healthful, however men suffering from issues with virility, can be clever to reduce the serving length and quantity. Some objects like alcohol and salty food will not high-quality lower virility, but is likewise horrible for the overall health and electricity so intake of these devices need to be accomplished only now and again. Processed meals and food devices which might be packed in plastic bins don't have any great dietary charge, and they're now not properly for fitness or virility. All guys involved with keeping best testosterone levels have to keep away from eating the ones virility-destroying substances.

Chapter 8: Testosterone Boosting Exercises

Most sorts of physical exertion can growth testosterone stages. Testosterone builds muscle, and with the ones clearly boosted levels, it does so right away[149]. In response to expanded bodily output, the frame copes thru growing the amount of testosterone secreted within the body. Because testosterone is a sturdy muscle builder, scrupulous athletes use injectable supplements of the hormone to construct bulk which has caused its banning in sports[150].

Aside from preservation of sexual trends in guys, testosterone is likewise important in body frame. Testosterone is an anabolic drug, that means it allows bulk up the body with the aid of developing muscle fibers and length[151]. This is why men with testosterone deficiency have lanky or overweight physiques (considering the truth that more fat bury the muscle groups) and document marked reduction in bodily and sexual normal average overall performance. Unfortunately, the amount of physical sports activities activities of human beings nowadays is substantially lower in contrast to the past a long term because of generation, behavior and leisure picks[152].

The proper statistics is there are physical sports activities that would dramatically decorate herbal testosterone degrees. It is specifically right that a few sports can beautify testosterone tiers. According to available proof from scientific studies, there are physical sports which can be observed to purpose an growth (or in a few, a drastic upward push) of serum testosterone. If achieved often, those sporting events can help hold a healthy dose of testosterone that can display beneficial in fixing many men's health proceedings.

According to research proper proper right here some excessive first-class physical physical video games are surely suitable in enhancing testosterone:

Sprinting

According to research, sprinting can considerably growth testosterone levels. The underlying mechanisms on how sprinting improves testosterone remains no longer absolutely understood. In a take a look at posted in Journal of Strength and Conditioning Research, handball gamers subjected to short sprint at the treadmill exhibited sizeable elevations of testosterone and extraordinary anabolic hormones (muscle-constructing hormones)[153].

Another test posted in International Journal of Sports Medicine hooked up that sprinting stepped forward plasma general testosterone[154]. It is also decided that doing repeated sprints at an growing and lowering distances (from 100 meters to 4 hundred meter, and vice versa) can growth testosterone in the bloodstream[155].

Sprinting is a traumatic physical hobby in phrases of power and power (capability to challenge strain short), and it calls for potential and exercise to sprint properly. But in evaluation to exclusive physical games, sprinting has no emphasis on physical staying power, which makes it an extremely good preference for beginners who're at the least acquainted the number one mechanism of this exercising[156]. Men interested by sprinting need to cautiously choose out a vicinity, ideally in good sized, litter-loose vicinity or specifically parks or sprinting tracks. Some recommended places encompass sprinting ovals in colleges, parks and in a tremendous unoccupied parking lots and empty hallways.

Lifting heavy weights

Weight-lifting is a extraordinary example of resistance education. In a resistance-type workout, the muscle fibers settlement in opposition to an out of doors strain (which consist of gravity)[157]. Lifting weights isn't always one-of-a-type to bodybuilders anymore; every person can carry out resistance training to decorate their testosterone levels. There are severa research helping the use of weights to improve testosterone tiers.

In have a have a take a look at located at the Journal of Applied Physiology, weight-lifting training for 10 weeks is tested to increase testosterone levels in more younger and older men – with older men (30-60 yrs) displaying more marked elevations[158]. Another comparable take a look at showed that acute resistance schooling additionally slightly improved testosterone tiers[159]. A paper published in the magazine Sports Medicine concluded that resistance physical games characterised thru immoderate volume protocols, slight and immoderate intensity, quick rest intervals and large muscle mass involvement have a tendency to provide finest will boom in testosterone and anabolic hormones like GH (growth hormone)[160]. Men who are weight knowledgeable will be predisposed to show off higher spikes in testosterone ranges throughout training classes[161]. Testosterone is also located to be a sturdy muscle builder that still inhibits protein degradation and heavy resistance workout is determined to result in acute will growth[162].

Studies show that heavy weights sporting activities are greater efficacious than lighter weights in growing testosterone levels inside the bloodstream. Start with dumbbells or kettle bells and educate at home. Increase intensity and weight gradually, ideally after training absolutely on a set weight for two weeks. Men looking for to bulk up, "lifting to exhaustion" sports are encouraged. Always have a check proper posture, and lift weights properly.

Tabata education

Tabata training is a version of high-intensity c programming language education (HIIT). HIIT is a quick but at the same time ridiculously robust exercise regular characterized thru bursts of extraordinarily extreme hobby intermingled with brief relaxation intervals[163]. HIIT is a totally excessive hobby and severa studies display that it is ideal for preserving and increasing testosterone levels.

In a have a look at posted in Journal of Applied Physiology, guys who're HIIT knowledgeable exhibited elevated testosterone stages in assessment to guys who exercised at low depth[164]. In every extraordinary comparable test, HIIT improves degrees of bloodstream testosterone and leptin[165] – leptin is a hormone that inhibits urge for meals for long time[166]. A look at posted in Journal of Endocrinological Investigation showed that HIIT physical activities helped increase unfastened testosterone as a nicely as channel it to androgen-sensitive tissues much like the muscular tissues and the gonads[167].

Let me say it directly – Tabata physical video video games are not smooth. However, HIIT or Tabata sports sports are confirmed immensely useful to testosterone and to physical common general overall performance. Tabata protocols with weight-lifting workout exercises also are well for developing muscle tone and elevating testosterone ranges[168]. Furthermore, HIIT may be finished in a great deal much less than 9 minutes! Tabata exercising exercises can be achieved the usage of a bounce rope, treadmill, motorcycle ergometer or perhaps "doing step ups" on stairs. A essential Tabata normal has 20 seconds of maximum bodily output (make as many repetitions as viable) located through way of a 10-second rest, and then repeat the entire regular eight times - for overall time of 4 minutes. Beginners must start with on 4 minute cycle, increasing to 2-4 cycles of a period of a few months.

Forced repetitions

Forced repetitions also are real for enhancing testosterone. Forced repetitions are basically overloading the muscle tissue to do more paintings beyond its perceived functionality. An instance of a forced repetition is at the same time as appearing a difficult and fast until exhaustion, the following and the next and very last rep is referred to as a pressured repetition. It is specially real that pressured repetitions push the body beyond perceived power. Not quality is this first rate for muscle constructing and power but moreover for maximizing testosterone production within the frame.

In a look at posted in International Journal of Sports Medicine, it determined that compelled repetitions exerted significantly greater will increase in testosterone degrees and neuromuscular responses in contrast to maximum repetitions[169]. A extraordinarily comparable have a examine published in Canadian Journal of Applied Physiology confirmed that forced repetitions can be advanced in elevating testosterone and increase hormone stages, even though every exercise routines confirmed will boom[170].

Forced repetitions have to be completed cleanly and efficiently, without 'cheating', for max gain. Forced repetitions also can be finished on lifting bodily video games - Just go through in mind these physical video games are greater susceptible to injuries in order that they'll want to be tried with more care. If completed frequently, pressured repetitions do emerge as simpler to carry out through the years.

Play (or watch) a competitive pastime

Playing sports activities sports activities may be a great manner to exercising and might prove a top notch testosterone booster, specifically if even as playing with surprising people. The huge intellectual stress that occurs at some point of a mainly intense wager or pastime will growth testosterone secretion, which builds up physical generic general performance.

Watching a notably aggressive exercising or match can also increase testosterone, so long as the institution supported wins. This is a double edged sword, as lower testosterone ranges can give up end result if the supporting group supported looses. Experts say that this mechanism is an evolutionary model designed to hurry up preparedness for a capability come upon and, after triumphing in competition to opponents, to put together for another bout of bodily contest – early people lived in a very competitive environment and we all have herbal variations to help us with aggressive situations. There are numerous research showing that excessive competitiveness (which best takes region whilst executed toward strangers) is also a huge testosterone booster.

In a have a have a examine among pistol-capturing game enthusiasts, assessments display that opposition has a unethical to (excuse the pun) shoot up testosterone degrees[171]. In each exclusive have a take a look at on basketball game enthusiasts, the volume of involvement in a quite aggressive challenge is correlated with testosterone tiers[172]. For the fanatics looking a televised game, the individuals whose group has received exhibited better testosterone levels in comparison to supporters of the dropping institution[173]. In a completely ultra-modern have a take a look at amongst rugby players posted in Journal of Strength and Conditioning Research, winning video games is associated with extended testosterone within the bloodstream[174].

To enhance testosterone, it's miles important to attempt to play greater aggressive employer video games, competitions or leagues for better exposure. For long time advantages it's miles constantly useful to take part in sports activities sports in which the maximum leisure is derived.

Chapter 9: Chopping firewood

A lumber axe may be the superb factor you want to growth herbal testosterone production. A brand new examine found out that act of decreasing wood causes upward spikes in testosterone ranges[175]. How it does so isn't simply understood, but experts postulated that it can be every distinctive evolutionary version for early people. Early humans just can't visit a supermarket to shop for food; they want to forage, hunt or do back-breaking agriculture to devour. The testosterone spikes is important in maintaining muscle tissues and strength in order that early human beings may additionally want to preserve their strength and lift a own family regardless of situations now not conducive to human existence.

Researchers from the University of California – Santa Barbara, studied a hard and fast of Tsimane tribesmen in the Amazon areas of Bolivia to look if non-competitive activities have any impact on testosterone levels. They sampled and as compared salivary testosterone degrees earlier than and after playing football and reducing wood. They determined out that cutting wooden improved testosterone degrees with the beneficial useful resource of as thousands as forty eight.6%! Compare that to spending time playing football which progressed testosterone to pleasant 17%. These consequences aren't affected by age or self-mentioned illness.

If you're lucky to have a rural area with masses of wood or lumber to cut or a cottage out inside the woods, its an top notch area to get an notable exercise and genuinely pump up testosterone (chop because it ought to be). Or, head to usa gala's and see if you'll be part of timber-reducing competitions there.

Have intercourse

In case you preferred to recognize, despite the fact that now not precisely defined as 'workout' or 'recreation', having sex is mounted to boom testosterone stages in men. Sexual interest is protected in this phase honestly because it (usually) consists of complete of existence bodily hobby.

In a have a look at on heterosexual couples, folks that truly had have sex exhibited fantastic will increase in testosterone[176]. In a observe on male purchasers in a sex membership, folks who watched sex acts exhibited 11% growth in testosterone at the same time as members have greater seventy % boom[177]. Furthermore, ejaculation after abstinence beginning from 7 to ten weeks is confirmed to motive high spikes in testosterone degrees in numerous studies[178][179].

Obviously, best have accountable sex with a consenting companion(s) and use good enough safety. You cannot enjoy your virility on the maximum if laid low with STD's, so continuously exercise steady sex.

Please take a look at safety even as exercise (or on the identical time as having intercourse)

The reader want to observe safety at the same time as exercising, and of direction at the same time as having intercourse. The essential rule in workout isn't always damage your self. Therefore, take a look at your device and surroundings earlier than use. Do no longer push yourself to the factor of self-harm. Remember that any damage will now not advantage your testosterone stages. In exercise, constantly apprehend your functionality and art work interior its limits. Keep in thoughts that on the same time as you are injured, it isn't always possible to workout well. Always wear right protective exercise device and function a have a look at safety rules. As with eating, if planning on having sex, obtain this responsibly.

Some physical sports proper here would possibly display genuinely tedious to do. It's understandable. Testosterone deficiency should make your muscle organizations fatigue fast, it certainly is disincentive to maintain exercise. My recommendation here is to begin small and then increase depth of exercises little by little. Start at a element most comfortable and then slightly boom for extra assignment every week. Motivation builds up from small successes, grade by grade at a time.

Testosterone Boosting Herbs

In this phase, the diverse herbs and spices which have shown to beautify testosterone degrees can be cited. Not excellent do many studies display that those herbs can obviously growth testosterone stages, however moreover decorate sexual average overall performance and virility. Some of these herbs are even historically regarded as aphrodisiacs.

Here are the listing of herbs verified to improve testosterone degrees in men:

Tongkat ali (Eurycoma longifolia)

A plant local in South East Asian international locations like Malaysia, Indonesia and Thailand, Tongkat Ali is traditionally touted as a sexual popular performance enhancer in men. Folklore medication calls for Tongkat Ali root in remedy of infertility, impotence and malaria, fatigue and tension. In modern, the sexual improving electricity of Tongkat Ali is supported thru research, wherein it's miles shown to assist boom testosterone tiers. In male rats, Tongkat Ali helped notably decorate male sexual behaviour in sexually-receptive girls, in addition to charge of spermatogenesis and sperm counts[180][181][182][183].

For human character person men Tongkat Ali can also moreover assist decorate testosterone ranges and control of past due-onset hypogonadism, in keeping with a test posted within the magazine Andrologia[184]. According to a have a take a look at posted in Asian Journal of Andrology, Tongkat Ali is placed powerful in improving sperm incredible and fertility in men with idiopathic infertility which can be associated with its impact on testosterone stages[185]. In a examine published in Evidence-Based Complementary and Alternative Medicine, Tongkat Ali proven to prevent and manage osteoporosis in men due to androgen deficiency, which suggests that the herb has a awesome impact on testosterone degrees inside the body[186]. These research are most effective a small choice of the severa research that have tested Tongkat Ali to be a remarkable herb which has a profound excessive satisfactory effect on male testosterone.

Tongkat Ali is to be had in nutritional dietary supplements. In such nutritional nutritional dietary supplements, Tongkat ali root powder is packed indoors drugs for oral intake. There are also some dietary supplements that blend Tongkat Ali with one-of-a-kind herbs. According to investigate, a hundred mg -three hundred mg of Tongkat ali root powder consistent with day for at the least one month can end end result to big changes in testosterone and virility.

Ginseng

Ginseng is a medicinal herb that is very well-known in East Asia, and is now gaining recognition in Western international locations. Ginseng root is historically applied in East Asian treatment to beautify highbrow and bodily normal overall performance, as well as improving male virility[187]. Today, Ginseng is likewise appeared to be well in boosting the immune tool and reducing blood sugar tiers[188]. There are severa research achieved which verify ginseng's ability to manifestly decorate testosterone in the body.

In a take a look at in rats, ginseng is determined to improve serum testosterone ranges[189]. Red ginseng given to rats additionally shows the equal effect, and it moreover improves spermatogenesis or manufacturing of sperm cells in keeping with a have a take a look at posted in Journal of Ginseng Research[190]. Human studies additionally show that ginseng helped improve unfastened and plasma testosterone, which guide its historical use as male reproductive aid[191]. According to a have a observe posted within the journal Endocrine Abstracts, ginseng may also even increase testosterone stages in girls[192]. There are already severa research displaying that ginseng may be useful for men with erectile disorder, which indicates that it can have an effect on serum testosterone[193]. Thus, ginseng also can show to be an first rate herb for enhancing testosterone ranges.

In Asian international locations, roots of ginseng are frequently visible bought entire and dried, or soaked in wine. Ginseng is likewise available in powder form. Some dietary dietary supplements additionally have ginseng as an active element. Dosages of ginseng variety from 500 mg to 3000 mg of dried root powder consistent with day for up to a few months. Always take ginseng preparations with food to keep away from belly disillusioned.

Maca root

Maca root is significantly to be had in dietary supplements. Historically, Maca root is used by historical South American cultures as a immoderate-altitude vegetable and as a prized aphrodisiac[194]. Maca root is concept to decorate sexual function consistent with severa research, which suggests that it is able to have an effect on testosterone metabolism.

Extracts from Maca root helped decorate sexual overall performance in male rats, consistent with a have a take a look at published inside the magazine Urology[195]. Some human studies show that Maca root may not at once increase stages of testosterone within the frame[196]. However, studies show that Maca root is useful in improving sperm manufacturing and motility in men, parameters in which testosterone performs an crucial detail[197]. Studies display that Maca root can also enhance the testosterone receptors inside the body, which improves response at the hormone.

It is less hard to locate Maca root in dietary supplements in area of the whole root. It may be very tough to discover complete Maca root in countries in which it isn't always nearby, at the aspect of Peru. According to to be had proof, the dosage of Maca root powder is one 450 mg tablet 3 times a day. Always take Maca root powder nutritional dietary supplements with food to keep away from capability belly dissatisfied.

Ginger

Ginger is an all-round spice that is famous in lots of cuisines anywhere in the global. In addition to its aromatic fragrant scent and slight heat flavor, the rhizomes of ginger is recognized for having healing packages for conditions like nausea and vomiting after surgical treatment, morning illness and arthritis[198]. The root of ginger includes several bioactive additives, similarly to its volatile oils and phenol compounds which can also additionally furthermore make contributions to its healing homes[199]. There are present studies displaying that ginger can also enhance testosterone production in guys.

Ginger helped enhance testosterone production in the testes of rats, and may additionally have protective results from the testicular toxicity exerted with the useful resource of lead[200]. Ginger even helped beautify testosterone manufacturing in rats with diabetes[201]. Addition of L-carnitine in ginger additionally seems to improve sexual overall performance in male rats[202]. These studies display that ginger is beneficial and beneficial in improving testosterone ranges inside the body.

It is viable to eat ginger in its complete shape. Add quantities of ginger to sautéed dishes for an Asian taste. Ginger can also be used as an fragrant aspect in smoothies. For dietary supplements containing ginger powder, 250 mg 4 times a day is consistent. For nutritional nutritional dietary supplements, usually take ginger with food to keep away from stomach infection.

Velvet bean (Mucuna pruriens)

Also known as cowhage, cowitch or cow-itch plant, or itch bean this little-stated herb grows in Africa, India and Caribbean global locations. The medical name of Velvet bean, Mucuna pruriens, is derived from the Latin phrase 'prurio' this means that 'itch'. The bean is located in the furry bean pod of the plant. The leaves and the hairy seed pod can motive extreme itching at the same time as touched. Historically, velvet bean were used in historic Chinese and Ayurvedic medicinal drug for the remedy of arthritis, involved issues and male reproductive troubles.

There are gift research showing that velvet bean can also enhance testosterone tiers within the body, which offers resource to its historical use as an aphrodisiac. In the mag African Journal of Biotechnology, an check showed that velvet bean extract added on first rate growth in testosterone ranges and weight of testes, prostate and seminal vesicles in rats[203]. According to any other examine positioned in The Journal of Sexual Medicine, velvet bean extract additionally helped boom testosterone tiers and sperm production in diabetic male rats[204]. In humans, the velvet bean has been mounted to be useful for infertile men on pinnacle of factors of strain and in phrases of sperm extraordinary which shows that it could have an up-regulating impact to testosterone degrees[205]. Another related have a look at on infertile guys published inside the magazine Fertility and Sterility showed that velvet bean undoubtedly expanded degrees of testosterone, luteinizing hormone and adrenalin in the serum, similarly to enhancing sperm counts and motility.

Velvet bean moreover has levodopa and serotonin, and hundreds of extra bioactive compounds[206]. Velvet bean has computer graphics apart from enhancing testosterone, so ensure to invite your doctor so it will not intervene with unique drugs. Velvet bean is frequently powdered and provided in supplements.

Cinnamon

Cinnamon is a very well-known spice that could be a well-known flavoring in baked items. Cinnamon is one of the few spices set up to help enhance testosterone tiers. Several studies assist the testosterone-boosting homes of cinnamon.

Diabetes has the tendency of decreasing testosterone levels in the frame. Cinnamon with ginger has showed to help enhance fertility, stepped forward serum insulin and testosterone in diabetic laboratory rats[207][208][209]. Even while administered by myself to rats, cinnamon additionally improves testosterone stages and sperm profiles[210]. Cinnamon additionally served protecting to the male reproductive organs in competition to toxicity because of the poison carbon tetrachloride, steady with a have a examine posted in the magazine Andrologia[211]. These studies really guide the capability of extracts in cinnamon to raise testosterone degrees.

Cinnamon is a spice significantly available in most global locations. Cinnamon is exceptional ate up through sprinkling it on baked items, or on liquids which includes espresso or in dairy primarily based definitely drinks which includes eggnog and malted milk.

Chapter 10: Testosterone Boosting Vitamins & Supplements

There are many supplements in the marketplace categorised to enhance sexual universal performance in guys. Some supplement compounds can enhance testosterone in combination with improving male sexual overall standard performance. We will speak some of the want to-have dietary supplements for guys, consistent with helping studies and clinical studies. Most of those elements may be determined in your close by health food or supplement store. Studies display that those dietary supplements are not best useful in increasing testosterone degrees, but moreover useful in enhancing male sexual enhancement.

Creatine

Creatine is a popular fitness supplement often used by bodybuilders and athletes to enhance athletic average typical performance. That's because of the reality Creatine is a natural muscle builder and serves as a gasoline deliver for the muscle agencies all through exercising. Creatine is likewise sincerely produced in the body. There are studies showing the advantages of additional supplementation of Creatine.

In addition to growing lean muscle groups and decreasing fat, Creatine is validated to significantly beautify serum testosterone in exercising guys as compared to placebo in keeping with a observe featured in International Journal of Sport Nutrition and Exercise Metabolism[212]. Another check posted in Clinical Journal of Sport Medicine used a double-blind placebo-managed crossover examine to determine if Creatine has any effect on testosterone, and discovered out that 3-week supplementation extended the degrees of DHT (dihydrotestosterone) in the serum[213]. DHT is the extra energetic form of testosterone this is without problem used inside the body, and in a BMJ study, higher ranges are correlated with superior quantity of weekly orgasms in men[214].

There are masses of dietary nutritional dietary supplements that encompass Creatine. There also are some dietary nutritional dietary supplements containing a natural shape of Creatine. Take be aware that Creatine is absorbed and fast metabolized within the body, so it's far crucial to comply with a consistent agenda for maximum appropriate outcomes. Creatine dosages are divided into 'loading' and 'protection' dose. The loading Creatine dose is 20 g-25g in keeping with day for 1 week, observed through safety dose of five g/day for two weeks[215].

DHEA

DHEA or Dehydroepiandrosterone is definitely a frame hormone that serves as a precursor to male and lady hormones[216]. DHEA is now found in numerous supplement preparations. DHEA degrees simply drops by the point we're past 30 years of age. This may also moreover provide an reason behind the slow good buy of intercourse hormones at some point of developing vintage. Chronic ailments moreover have a propensity to reduce DHEA stages in the frame; in a check among diabetic men with excessive serum insulin ranges, low DHEA is also associated with low testosterone[217]. There are greater studies below displaying the affiliation among DHEA and testosterone.

Supplementation of 3 hundred mg DHEA is decided to beautify sexual arousal in postmenopausal women, which may be due to expanded response of testosterone[218]. In men, supplementation of DHEA enabled sufferers with erectile disease to have progressed erection sufficient for sexual hobby[219]. DHEA severe approximately the resource of mouth moreover helped substantially growth testosterone tiers in male volunteers[220].

Even in spite of the truth that DHEA is already produced in our our bodies, studies display that we will benefit from greater supplementation. For DHEA-containing dietary nutritional dietary supplements, without a doubt take it with meals.

DHEA may want to engage with tablets which includes insulin, anastrozole, exemestane and fulvestrant, and medicinal tablets metabolized within the liver which incorporates lovastatin, ketoconazole, itraconazole, fexofenadine and triazolam and masses of others. Do ask your medical doctor if taking DHEA is consistent and will not engage with prescribed drug treatments.

L-arginine

L-arginine is also a famous complement. L-arginine is actually a type of amino acid that still takes place to be produced inside the frame. Because it's far an amino acid, L-arginine is also observed in protein-wealthy meals[221]. Men trying to enhance sexual primary overall performance need to take greater L-arginine. L-arginine is an critical precursor to nitric oxide[222]. Nitric oxide is a compound with essential biologic functions within the human body, and its number one effect is to dilate blood vessels and act as a neurotransmitter among nerve cells[223]. For men, nitric oxide plays a critical role inside the erection of the penis[224]. Therefore, low nitric oxide levels manner your penis will erect an awful lot much less frequently and insufficiently hard at some point of intercourse[225].There are studies showing that L-arginine supplementation can in all likelihood remedy sexual ordinary overall performance troubles in men.

In an test on rats, management of L-arginine stepped forward testicular blood go with the glide (higher nourishment and function) and nitrous oxide degrees in wholesome rats[226]. Mice fed with L-arginine terrible food plan exhibited decrease testosterone stages[227]. Human research additionally showed that supplementation of L-arginine helped lower blood pressure in hypertensive people; this effect can be due to increased nitric acid manufacturing elicited via L-arginine[228][229]. This action of L-arginine to blood pressure is vital due to the reality it's far understood that hypertension can reason erectile sickness[230].

Optimum blood pressure is wanted so blood can float more without difficulty into the penis and cause erection. Because nitric oxide dilates the arteries, more blood can flow into the penis and outcomes to stronger and longer-lasting erections. This makes L-arginine a have to-have supplement for men. Illnesses and pressure have bad results on nitric oxide degrees within the body, so supplementation of L-arginine can be essential.

The dose range of L-arginine is 6 to 30 grams consistent with day. Keep in thoughts that L-arginine can increase or extend the effects of blood pressure- and ldl ldl cholesterol-decreasing medicinal pills. Like in DHEA, ask your doctor earlier than taking L-arginine dietary dietary dietary supplements to save you any unfavourable drug interactions.

Zinc

Zinc is an vital mineral this is critical for the human frame[231]. Zinc is needed for correct mobile metabolism, immune device function and making proteins, wound restoration and developing DNA and cell branch. Zinc is also very essential in guys's health, and severa studies display that it is able to decorate testosterone and fertility.

Zinc plays an crucial element in sexual everyday performance and advanced testosterone tiers, in keeping with a check in male rats posted in the Journal of Reproductive Sciences[232]. Optimum stages of zinc is important to reproductive function in guys regular with a take a look at posted in Indian Journal of Pathology and Microbiology, that men with fertility troubles tend to have terrible ranges of the mineral[233]. Adequate degrees of zinc are related to sperm motility, and coffee stages are associated with subfertility and unexplained infertility[234][235]. In men with fertility problems, more zinc for 3 months progressed testosterone ranges, DHT degrees and sperm counts, on the identical time as 9 higher halves (out of 22) have become pregnant[236].

Zinc is incredible taken orally, sixty six milligrams consistent with day for 26 weeks consistent with Mayo Clinic[237]. Zinc may be involved about meals to save you stomach disappointed.

Vitamin D

Vitamin D is a fat-soluble diet and an crucial nutrient. Vitamin D strengthens bones and the immune system, and essentially prolongs existence[238]. Because of its advantages, nutrition D is one of the famous vitamins fortified in processed substances. In order to be healthy, men require good enough additives of vitamins D[239]. There are severa outstanding studies displaying that nutrients D can assist decorate sexual average general overall performance and reproductive fulfillment in guys.

Testicular characteristic is associated with appropriate enough stores of weight-reduction plan D and deficiency may additionally additionally moreover quit result to problems in production of sperm cells and androgens, whilst good enough tiers is related to more effective reproductive achievement consistent with research in rats[240][241][242]. Adequate food plan D stages are associated with higher stages of testosterone in men, regular with a have a have a examine featured in Clinical Endocrinology[243]. Men with low testosterone degrees regularly have horrible nutrition D in the serum, in step with a present day take a look at posted in the European Journal of Endocrinology[244]. In addition, men who have negative testosterone and low vitamins D stages face better hazard of loss of life from cardiovascular and non-cardiovascular troubles (making nutrients D a lifesaver simply)[245]. Low weight-reduction plan D ranges moreover will increase predisposition to erectile disorder[246]. The abundance of sunshine may provide an explanation for why reproductive success is better in summer time months than in winter[247].

In experiments in hairless rats, good enough weight loss program D supplementation superior hair boom[248]. Furthermore, men and women with ok nutrients D degrees have a propensity to have lower frame fat content material cloth cloth[249][250]. In addition to improving natural testosterone ranges and male virility, nutrition D allows keep healthy frame weight (regardless of the reality that extra supplementation isn't probable to reason brilliant weight loss[251]).

Despite its time period due to the fact the 'sunshine healthy eating plan', records indicates that many human beings virtually be by poor food plan D in line with a have a study featured in The American Journal of Clinical Nutrition [252]. Even good enough solar publicity (as a minimum 1.Five hours/week, or 12.Eighty 5 mins/day) is not any assure to prevent nutrients D deficiency[253]. In a have a observe among East Asians in Australia (which has tropical to temperate climate), factors which encompass greater sun-safety behaviour and much less mins of solar exposure in weekends already increase risk of eating regimen D deficiency. Vitamin D deficiency is apparent even within the United States, it truly is sudden due to the truth many processed components on this united states of america are fortified with the weight loss program[254]. Living further from the equator, having darker skin and being overweight are crucial elements to recollect at the same time as it comes figuring out if there's a deficiency of food regimen D[255][256].

All of this facts suggests the importance of weight loss plan D now not just for appropriate sexual and reproductive overall performance, but additionally for fundamental health. Even eating fortified food and basking in daytime isn't always sufficient to prevent eating regimen D deficiency. Therefore, men have to have weight-reduction plan D dietary supplements for improvement of testosterone and sexual usual performance. The each day requirement of nutrition D in guys is minimum 600 IU, and older human beings might also moreover need as a whole lot as 800 IU[257]. Men with poor diet regime D ranges may also moreover want to have eight,400 IU regular with week for 3 weeks.

Vitamin E

Vitamin E some extraordinary fats-soluble eating regimen with mentioned antioxidant homes[258]. There are several kinds of vitamins E, with alpha-tocopherol the maximum strong and nutritionally useful to the human frame[259]. Vitamin E is observed in severa common elements, but most effective in lots a lot much less extremely good form of gamma-tocopherol[260]. According to research, there can be evidence that more supplementation of diet E can assist guys with fertility problems[261].

Supplementation of food plan E with selenium helped beautify sperm motility and morphology in sub-fertile men[262]. In a have a take a look at posted in Archives of Andrology, men with fertility issues who took vitamins E plus selenium for 3 months additionally exhibited lower oxidation markers and better sperm motility[263]. In a huge test published in International Journal of General Medicine, Infertile men who took weight loss plan E and selenium for at least a hundred days exhibited better semen remarkable, sperm motility and morphology, and 10.Eight% extended expenses of spontaneous being pregnant in comparison to men with out a treatment[264]. This suggests that nutrients E and selenium are a want to-have complement for guys with fertility troubles.

Because it could increase manufacturing of LH (luteinizing hormone) and FSH (follicle stimulating hormone), and the protecting impact to Leydig cells within the testicles, weight loss plan E might also moreover play a feature for pinnacle of the street manufacturing of testosterone[265][266]. Furthermore, more nutrients E supplementation may additionally reduce the chance of prostate most cancers in men who smoke tobacco[267].

Even despite the fact that there are not any research showing that weight loss program E can enhance libido or sexual performance, its benefits are too huge for men to brush aside. Except in nuts and seed oils, the amount of weight loss program E in meals is low so supplementation is wanted. For guys, the advocated dosage of nutrients E is eighty to 100 mcg a day; the most solid dose is hundred mcg a day.

Magnesium

Magnesium is a hint and important mineral with severa organic roles within the human frame. Magnesium is an electrolyte, a neurotransmitter and is critical in making enzymes, so it placed in all cells. Low stages of magnesium within the bloodstream can result in many specific fitness problems. In men, magnesium plays an important function in testosterone and proper function of the reproductive device.

In an take a look at in rats, magnesium-wealthy water helped improve shape and feature of the testicles and serum testosterone tiers[268]. Magnesium can also moreover enhance the producing of testosterone after exercise in athletes and sedentary humans, with exercise individuals gaining more increase[269]. Furthermore, management of magnesium may moreover growth the frame's capability to apply testosterone inside the bloodstream[270]. This can offer an reason for the consequences of an check in which supplementation of zinc and magnesium advanced testosterone and strength tiers in athletes versus placebo, constant with a have a examine posted in Journal of Exercise Physiology[271]. In a look at posted in International Journal of Andrology, testosterone and insulin boom element (which enlarges muscle fibers and strengthens bone) stages are independently associated with serum selenium and magnesium stages in older guys[272].

Magnesium may additionally moreover play a small function in fertility. There is a small association amongst low magnesium and zinc tiers and malformed sperm cells, consistent with a test published in Reproductive Toxicology[273]. Since magnesium is a neurotransmitter, it could play a element within the pathology of premature ejaculation; the muscle organizations that manipulate ejaculation are managed thru magnesium-containing neurotransmitters. Two research already showed that guys affected by untimely ejaculation will be predisposed to have low magnesium tiers in the bloodstream[274][275].

The studies show that men need to have most appropriate magnesium degrees to stay bodily robust, have nicely testosterone stages and live longer in mattress, and be able to impregnate and feature children. This moreover manner that men need to have adequate shops of magnesium of their our our our bodies due to the fact the semen has excessive magnesium stages. For this motive, magnesium supplementation is vital in sexually-active guys.

Magnesium levels generally generally tend to drop even as guys devour alcohol, have bouts of diarrhea and whilst the use of diuretics, or maybe at the same time as sweating profusely. Since an entire lot of food are not proper assets of this mineral, men have to take dietary supplements with magnesium, most proper four hundred-420 mg consistent with day[276].

L-carnitine

L-carnitine is an amino acid that has antioxidant residences. L-carnitine is likewise a well-known supplement frequently advertised as a fats burner. It has foundation because of the reality L-carnitine permits delivery fatty acids to the cell mitochondria (powerhouse of the mobile) to provide energy. Doctors are also conscious that L-carnitine is useful for patients with excessive cardiovascular problems together with angina, coronary coronary coronary heart attack and coronary coronary heart failure and peripheral vascular sickness, even though how it exactly works in those times isn't always properly understood. There remains plenty to learn about the coolest consequences of L-carnitine inside the body, however there are already studies displaying that it is beneficial to guys with erectile sickness, infertility and awful sperm profile, and Peyronie's contamination.

There is proof that L-carnitine is useful for men with early-diploma and acute Peyronie's illness i.E. Penile curvature and deformity in a few unspecified time in the destiny of erection[277]. In some one of a kind study, L-carnitine with verapamil helped lessen penile curvature and drift in men with superior and resistant Peyronie's sickness[278]. L-carnitine is likewise useful for men with erection problems, specifically while administered with drugs like sildenafil and vardenafil. In research, L-carnitine administered with erectile disease drugs proved extra efficacious than even as drugs have been given by myself[279][280].

In a take a look at in male hemodialysis sufferers, low L-carnitine degrees are correlated to depressed free testosterone degrees[281]. This indicates that L-carnitine moreover plays a feature in sexual overall performance in guys. This is supported via a Urology check wherein men supplemented with L-carnitine similarly exhibited higher erections and frequency of nocturnal erections in preference to placebo, and suspension resulted to reversal of those benefits[282]. Another present day observe confirmed that guys with negative intercourse force who took L-carnitine with L-arginine and ginseng reported better sexual satisfaction and better sperm tendencies profile in evaluation to placebo[283].

However, the first-class impact of L-carnitine might be on improving fertility. L-carnitine is present inside the semen, and severa research research show that higher values are correlated with greater numbers of more healthful sperm cells[284][285][286][287]. The feature of L-carnitine in semen isn't certainly understood, but a test in cows wherein it's far proven that L-carnitine helped beautify sperm survival and motility as quickly because it entered the girl reproductive tract[288]. When given to infertile subjects, L-carnitine helped boom sperm rely, motility and morphology although an appropriate mechanism but stays unexplained[289][290]. In a take a look at published in Journal of Assisted Reproduction and Genetics, L-carnitine even helped decorate sperm tendencies in men who smoke[291].

According to these numerous studies, guys should generally take nutritional dietary supplements of L-carnitine for added virility. Men with lingering fertility troubles because of bad semen remarkable derive the most advantage from L-carnitine supplementation. In studies, the impact of L-carnitine supplementation will become obvious after four to six months of non-prevent treatment. The endorsed dosage of L-carnitine can range from 500 mg to two grams in line with day.

Be careful on the same time as choosing dietary dietary supplements made for guys

There are severa nutritional supplements, herbs and spices offered at the net as nutritional supplements to decorate testosterone tiers. These can even be observed at many fitness-orientated internet sites and complement shops. We left out a whole lot of them in this e-book due to the fact there's no strong evidence that they might help boom testosterone levels.

Chapter 11: Testosterone Destroying Lifestyle Habits

Men essential approximately improving their testosterone simply want to be familiar with common manner of existence conduct which is probably diagnosed to damage testosterone. Many of these conduct are grossly horrific and may have an effect at the frame in more than one procedures - now not in reality reducing testosterone levels.

Sleep deprivation

Being deprived of sleep is one of the most common testosterone and libido killers. A man or woman without adequate sleep isn't always in splendid fitness. Sleep deprivation is massive, and it's basically making human beings sick. At least 50 to 70 million adults within the United States be anxious through way of sleep deprivation because of sleep troubles and wakefulness[292].

Many research studies display that sleep deprivation can boom infection inside the frame, weaken the immune tool, make us fats, diabetic, hypertensive and depressed[293]. Lack of sleep can give up cease end result to vehicle accidents, reduced cognitive abilties, heart illnesses and actually increases the risk of early death[294]. Furthermore, loss of sleep can badly injure men's virility in terms of testosterone ranges and sex power.

A have a take a look at published within the journal Sleep focusing on older men verified how standard sleep time predicts usual and loose testosterone levels[295]. In older guys, low testosterone degrees are also related to horrible sleep performance, improved frame weight and sleep disturbances which for which showed a strong link amongst testosterone and sleep[296].

In a examine featured in The Journal of American Medical Association, healthful younger guys subjected to 5 hours of sleep for each week professional 10% to 15% drop in sunlight hours testosterone levels[297]. In an test published inside the mag Biological

Psychiatry, it's far proven that sleep deprivation in particular reduced testosterone levels in guys[298].

The above referred to studies show that sleep extraordinary has a direct effect to intercourse hormones and sexual functioning. For men who find out that their average overall performance in bed is inside the rut, an awesome question to ask oneself is whether or not they may be getting enough best sleep. It is likewise important to look at out for sleep problem symptoms including snoring, lack of functionality to go to sleep at night time time and unusual vocalizations at the same time as asleep, falling asleep during sports, or uncommon urge to go to sleep at daylight hours. For those worried about their sleep styles, its an great idea to invite your companion or sleep mate (commonly they're likely extra reliable) for a few element uncommon at night time time. For those now not capable of acquire restful sleep, clinical assist for a capability sleep issues want to be taken into consideration.

Alcohol abuse

Alcohol is one of the handiest busters of virility and motives of low testosterone. Alcohol abuse lowers virility in men and motives bargain in sexual functioning, now not to mention consequences in making men bodily lots less appealing (for instance the "Beer Gut").

Alcohol is one of the maximum not unusual bodily motives of erectile ailment[299]. Even in men with apparently responsive erections, ingestion of an excessive amount of alcohol (binge consuming) can result in the inability to have or sustain an well tough erection for sex. Men who devour huge portions (greater than pictures or servings) of alcohol on a each day foundation or have the compulsion to drink, to drink on my own or conceal at the same time as consuming or experience withdrawal signs and symptoms while not ingesting - the ones are signs and signs of active alcoholism and negatively effects every natural testosterone manufacturing and virility[300].

Alcohol influences virility as it messes up with the mind (clouded questioning makes "appealing times" indiscernible) and could growth blood strain (increased blood stress makes it more tough to have an erection)[301].

Men who're alcoholics often have courtroom docket cases like untimely ejaculation, low sexual desire and erectile sickness, in line with a test on male topics in a cleaning middle[302]. Alcohol consumption is also positioned to be correlated with extraordinary erection mechanisms that make contributions to erectile disorder[303]. In a test amongst Chinese person grownup adult males, ingesting 3 or more elegant alcoholic liquids in keeping with week is validated to boom chance of sexual dissatisfaction and erectile sickness specially on individuals who smoke[304]. Still, how alcohol precisely messes with the mechanisms of penile erection isn't always clearly understood[305].

Alcohol is also horrible for testosterone and fertility. In animal experiments, alcohol is established to purpose shrinking of the testicles and prostate gland, and discount in testosterone degrees[306][307]. In guys acute alcoholic intoxication is confirmed to depress testosterone stages within the bloodstream, steady with a look at posted in The Journal of Pharmacology and Experimental Therapeutics[308]. This finding is replicated once more in a have a look at posted in the magazine Alcohol and Alcoholism, this time on each ladies and men[309]. In a few different test posted in Indian Journal of Physiology and Pharmacology, male alcoholics are placed to have decrease testosterone and impaired sperm motility, and the deficiency is more said in men with longer duration of alcohol abuse[310].

It can be real that alcohol may have the effect of increasing the opportunities of hooking up with someone else due to the fact ethanol reduces social inhibitions[311]. Still, there is greater proof showing that alcohol taken in greater is horrible for health and virility, even notwithstanding it illusionary outcomes. Men looking for to enhance their normal performance in bed want to reduce out the ones each day alcoholic liquids. Men showing behaviors along side; having a compulsion to drink, a want to cover consuming from others, feeling irritated even as the ritual alcohol is questioned or disturbed and preserve alcohol in places which includes automobile, paintings table or place of job, or have art work and dating problems because of ingesting, or have emotions of guilt approximately eating, need to bear in mind attempting to find professional help.

Tobacco

Another robust element that reduces virility is tobacco abuse. At least 21.6% of person men in the United States smoke cigarettes[312]. It is also crucial to understand that fifty % of those men moreover be afflicted via manner of erectile disease. Tobacco use is often viewed as a behavior associated with masculinity, bodily dominance or conduct. However studies display that the usage of tobacco products can take a toll on sexual normal performance, considerably on guys.

There are numerous studies displaying that tobacco may be horrible for guys's sexual average performance. Tobacco use can purpose persistent narrowing of the blood vessels in the frame, together with within the penis, which reasons erection problems in men regular with U.S. National Institutes of Health (NIH)[313]. Tobacco is a incredible promoter of erectile ailment. A look at in Urology confirmed that impotence is more large among people who smoke than in non-individuals who smoke[314]. In a take a look at featured in American Journal of Epidemiology, majority of erectile disorder patients have been located out to be present day individuals who smoke in particular on men a long term 50 and above, and men with history of smoking is at chance[315]. Along with cardiovascular illness, erectile disorder is a strongly related disease on smoking consistent with a evaluate of contemporary studies[316][317]. In each extraordinary populace-primarily based totally have a have a observe among guys in Boston place, cumulative multi-% years of smoking are related to erectile dysfunction; even passive smoking has shown an extended chance[318]. Despite early promotions and commercials suggesting that tobacco use improves masculinity, it does the opportunity because of the truth that it's far associated with erectile issues[319].

Tobacco also can affect testosterone stages, despite the fact that no longer right now. There are studies even displaying that male people who smoke have same or better testosterone tiers than non-folks who smoke[320]. Tobacco use may not decrease testosterone levels[321], however may additionally growth sex-hormone binding globulin (SHBG) ranges that lessen the quantity of testosterone that can be used by the frame[322].

Tobacco is likewise an essential predictor of male infertility[323]. In a have a observe featured in Fertility and Sterility, cigarette smokers exhibited reduced sperm counts, sperm motility and regular sperm counts in evaluation to non-smokers[324]. In an Asian Journal of Andrology have a observe on Chinese guys, medium-, heavy- and prolonged-term smokers in a fertility hospital moreover tested negative semen remarkable[325]. This finding is supported with the aid of some different have a examine on infertile men in which it is confirmed that smoking is one of the brilliant factors for terrible semen fantastic and sperm counts and viability that outcomes to infertility[326].

There are many one-of-a-kind research we did now not include but almost all of them say that tobacco use isn't beneficial for men's reproductive fitness. Those men who need to maintain or undo the harm due to smoking need to end the use of tobacco and avoid places in which smoking takes location. Quitting tobacco is a whole lot less hard with the assist of a medical physician and via enlisting the help from pals and family (who're ideally non-those who smoke).

Obesity

Obesity has an simple inverse affiliation with unfastened testosterone levels[327]. Even in boys present technique puberty, obese man or woman males usually usually generally tend to have decrease testosterone degrees in assessment to their leaner counterparts[328]. In a observe featured in the magazine Diabetes Care, it's far found out that forty% of obese non-diabetic guys and 50% of obese diabetic men have lower-than-everyday levels of testosterone[329]. In addition, weight problems and metabolic syndrome (weight troubles with excessive blood stress, blood sugar and ldl ldl ldl cholesterol) is known to growth danger of sexual illness in guys, particularly to those with diabetes[330].

Men with weight problems additionally face extra chance of erectile ailment, specially to guys with type-2 diabetes[331]. In a check among Danish guys published in Journal of Sexual Medicine, weight troubles is demonstrated to be associated with erectile sickness especially on extra younger guys age 20-45 years[332]. A in particular similar take a look at published in Journal of Andrology, this time on guys at a Navy Recruit Training Center, additionally concluded that popular weight problems is related to erectile disorder[333]. In a populace-primarily based surely test posted in European Journal of Clinical Endocrinology, it concluded that erectile illness is each normal in non-overweight guys with high frame mass (obese) and guys with weight problems[334].

Obesity moreover has an impact on the great of semen and sperm, in step with a have a look at in Reproductive Health.[335]. A examine posted in Fertility and Sterility showed that immoderate or very low frame mass index (BMI) is related to terrible semen awesome[336].

These research show how vital it's far for men to lose immoderate frame weight. Lose the spare tire and regain now not definitely out of region virility, however also self-confidence and further first-rate outlook. The splendid manner to shed pounds is to change lifestyle behavior; with the aid of slowly changing repeatable each day habits. Dieting is in no way a incredible solution for weight troubles because of the truth it is short and the out of place weight will genuinely be regained decrease again. Rather than food regimen, it's also ideal to discover opportunity, nutrient dense ingredients which may be amusing to devour and assemble this into a dependancy which may be sustained inside the course of one's whole lifestyles.

Chapter 12: Prolonged physical exertion or aerobic

This also can sound contradictory, but there can be proof that workout for prolonged durations (extra than an hour) can display a bane to testosterone. Long stretches of exercise in mild to moderate depth are frequently termed as 'cardio' or cardio workout. Some actual examples of aerobic exercising embody extended-distance strolling, swimming and rowing and marathons.

There are studies especially bringing up that aerobic exercising for prolonged intervals can harm testosterone. Some examples of prolonged cardio physical sports activities consist of prolonged-distance strolling, rowing, brisk walking and swimming.

According to a check published in Canadian Journal of Applied Physiology, rats who were made to swim for three hours for five days every week for 4 weeks exhibited shrinkage of testicles and discount in testosterone stages[337]. In some other similar have a look at in rats, 10 weeks of workout (four hours swim every day) markedly decreased testosterone and reproductive ability[338]. In a human study published in Journal of Applied Physiology, members subjected to enormous aerobic exercise exhibited lower testosterone degrees as compared to those who did no longer finished any workout[339]. Aerobic and anaerobic workout is not tested to boom testosterone degrees 2 hours after exercise, in line with each different human have a look at posted in Journal of Sports Sciences[340]. Even elite runners experience both no trade or a decline in testosterone stages after a semi-persistence run, constant with a Asian Journal of Sports Medicine test[341]. A prolonged-term take a look at confirmed that guys who enrolled in a one year-prolonged slight-depth cardio software program did not showcase extended testosterone levels[342]. Sedentary men additionally did not gain any testosterone gain from twelve weeks of aerobics and low-frequency exercising, consistent with a test posted in Central European Journal of Public Health[343].

Testosterone degrees have a tendency to drop after a specifically lengthy bodily hobby (greater than 2 hours) due to the fact androgens interfere with frame mechanisms that restore broken muscle fibers, bring about muscle-fiber hypertrophy and muscle-harm rehabilitation[344]. Testosterone forces the muscle organizations to perform better, and in doing so, prevents harm restore. By scaling decrease back testosterone degrees after extended exertion, the battered muscle agencies are allowed get higher.

It is not accurate to say that aerobic exercising is terrible for the body. Aerobics is right in enhancing muscular reaction, lowering blood stress and in causing modest weight reduction. But if the goal is to enhance testosterone ranges, doing aerobics for extra than an hour won't display beneficial. Other types of cardio exercise include dancing exercises, tennis, biking, ergometer and elliptical instructor. It continues to be feasible to carry out those wearing sports , so long as they will be not for extended durations of time - preferably plenty much less than an hour at a time. Save greater time with the beneficial aid of doing Tabata as an alternative; it most effective takes four-6 mins and is a lot higher for boosting herbal testosterone.

Psychological pressure

Immense and common mental strain is likewise stated to cause issues in virility in guys. Immense pressure can also make stress down sexual preference. Some common mental stresses embody despair, tension, records of bodily, emotional, or sexual abuse, pressure and fatigue and terrible verbal exchange or conflict with a romantic companion.

Specifically, depression and tension are related to erectile disease[345][346].This is a state of affairs due to the fact depressive and anxiety issues are amazing. In addition there are numerous reasons and belongings of pressure and masses of them cannot be avoided. There are many research linking pressure to erectile disease.

Men with put up-disturbing stress sickness (PTSD) regularly have poorer sexual general overall performance, especially individuals who are gift method remedy; sexual disorder is a commonplace detrimental impact of hysteria drug treatments[347]. Depressed men additionally generally have a tendency to be bothered via erectile sickness, and treatment with sildenafil helped beautify depressive signs and symptoms[348]. This is supported with the aid of manner of a Journal of Sexual Medicine test demonstrating that ED related appreciably with depression and tension reputation in middle-aged Japanese men[349]. In flip erectile disorder also can count on anxiety and melancholy in more youthful guys, in step with a have a look at posted in Journal of Sex and Marital Therapy[350]. In addition, low testosterone degrees increase chance of having melancholy, anxiety and decreased first-class of existence, which may be ameliorated through manner of greater supplementation in line with a have a look at posted in Endocrine Journal[351].

It is likewise a trouble that severa drugs for remedy of hysteria and melancholy can reason erectile disease and lack of hobby in sexual sports. However, this is not a cause to forego remedy for tension and depression. Most docs are very aware of this trouble and they are capable of help regain sexual function and virility at the identical time as present way treatment.

Everyone memories pressure and positive tiers of mental anxiety, however the threshold termed as demanding differs among humans. For instance, work-associated very last dates can also show stressful to your co-employee but not to you. Simply staying far from strain won't be the realistic solution. First, it is vital as a way to discover the statistics that reasons pressure. Second, it is also vital to are seeking out for help from highbrow stress. Sexual dysfunction (erectile troubles, low libido, and plenty of others.) as a result of strain method that there may be already a toll on your health and may even need expert help. Self-medicating and coping is normally not enough to clear up mental pressure. The common treatment modalities for mental stress frequently do now not contain manage of medication. Most specialists stick to speak treatment, relaxation schooling and strain control and ache coping capabilities in treating mental pressure, and having the ones remedies assist remedy sexual or erectile disorder.

Chapter 13: Testosterone, a completely unique hormone

A short records

The troubles and ability interests raised by way of using a loss of testosterone aren't new. We locate, from -1300 BC, passages evoking the castration of Chinese officers. For the imperial authorities, this approach had the gain of submitting the mission and stopping any hazard of insurrection, and it became systematically devoted till 1912. Tens of lots of eunuchs had been as a end result "fortunate" to be retained as administrators, a position whose importance has been confirmed on severa sports for the duration of information [1].

The Normans, on their issue, did no longer hesitate to punish an overly belligerent rival via imposing on him castration and dismantling. As for women from a wealthy social historical past, they desired to preserve relationships and sexual favors with castrated slaves, the principle advantage being the almost nil chance of being pregnant. Docility, hairless frame and non-existent fertility: those are already the issue effects of a completely low testosterone degree skilled with the beneficial useful resource of people, no matter the fact that cutting-edge-day treatment did now not but exist. To reduce down them, Pliny the Elder recommended the intake of animal testicles - the start of the problem end up mentioned from Antiquity.

If a few progress is recorded ultimately of present day-day-day times, it's miles round the second one half of the 19th century that we begin to completely apprehend the outcomes of castration in animals. Colloquiums were prepared, with the end result of some thrilling clinical advances however regardless of the fact that now not very convincing.

It have become not till the twelve months 1935 that a hard and fast of researchers led with the resource of Ernst Laqueur isolated testosterone and made this discovery public -

estrogen had been isolated as early as 1929. Then started out a period dubbed the "golden age of steroid chemistry ", characterized through a achievement experiments and essential advances.

Since then, research have followed one another: there had been 256 in 1956, greater than one thousand in 1976. Today, they're now not counted. This research has enabled us to apprehend the a couple of underlying mechanisms of testosterone, so much in order that currently, few secrets and techniques and strategies stay. However, it is easy that too few people are definitely privy to the ability effects of testosterone, if no longer through the contribution of stereotypes and preconceived thoughts. It is time to dig deeper.

Welcome to biology magnificence

It's tough to write down any such guide with out talking about testosterone as an entire. As a steroid and androgenic hormone, it's miles liable for sexual functioning and reproductive mechanisms. The testes in guys and, to a lesser volume, the ovaries in women are the principle producers of testosterone, with the adrenal glands and surrounding tissues playing handiest a minor characteristic.

Globally, it's far anticipated that men have 7 to eight instances extra testosterone than women: this inequality is defined through a better hormonal exposure within the route of pregnancy [2].

When testosterone is produced and circulates in the blood, it binds to diverse unique plasma shipping proteins, the primary one being SHGB - Sex hormone-binding globulin. Likewise, a part of the circulating testosterone is transformed into estrogen: that is the technique of aromatization. Only unfastened testosterone, ie neither fine nor converted, is to be had to the frame.

If generating loads of testosterone is the favored impact, the frame need with the intention to dispose of it freely! Changes in way of life, particularly via food plan and exercise, are sometimes enough to beautify this parameter.

Furthermore, it's miles vital to word that testosterone ranges aren't solid: higher in the morning, they typically generally tend to lower because of the fact the day progresses. If you want to recognize your hormonal reputation, it's miles critical to have a blood test spherical 10 a.M., preferably on an empty belly. Normal testosterone values for individual men are among 264-916 ng / dL, but might also range counting on the reference laboratory [3].

Finally, permit's mention the number one active by-product of testosterone: dihydrotestosterone, shortened DHT. Resulting from a partial conversion of testosterone, DHT has fantastically similar homes. It is mainly responsible for pubertal sexual differentiation (musculature, hairiness, sexual improvement) and increased fertility. Some researchers have moreover highlighted its hyperlink with alopecia, no matter the reality that this claim stays debated [4].

These short prolegomena have allowed us to have a examine a bit bit more approximately the herbal form of testosterone. The number one aspect then remains: the capability consequences of testosterone at the frame. Numerous and occasionally outstanding, it's miles essential to apprehend them at the way to higher apprehend the effects of hormonal variations.

The effects of testosterone on the Human Body

The human body is without issues malleable. Never steady, it is continuously subjected to one of a kind organic variations. High tiers of testosterone can because of this bring about sturdy modifications, even after puberty: libido, temper, fatigue, muscle improvement ... These outcomes can't - and want to now not - be underestimated.

Fetal improvement and puberty

The movement of testosterone begins offevolved even in advance than begin: it will initiate sexual differentiation, determine future androgenic sensitivity and alter the morphology of the unborn toddler [5]. DHT and different steroid hormones also play a key role in this revealing way.

Puberty is the second essential step in an character's bodily and hormonal transformation. Around age eleven, the hypothalamus step by step will boom its production of GnRH (gonadotropin releasing hormone), main to an increase in LH (luteinizing hormone) and FSH (follicle stimulating hormone). These molecules will subsequently motive a full-size rise in testosterone.

Sexual differentiation is then accentuated even extra: the beard grows, the pores and skin thickens, the fat mass decreases, pimples appears ... The outcomes can hold till adulthood.

Muscles

Testosterone is the deliver of muscle boom and protection, irrespective of age. Studies have proven that administering testosterone to poor men effects in decreased preferred weakness, improved electricity and stamina, and most significantly, muscle fiber development [6]. A excessive percent of lean frame mass is consequently correlated with a immoderate testosterone level, and this explains the variations in frame composition located amongst males and females.

Various studies have supported this finding, and characteristic confirmed that, as an example, men with prostate cancer had a decrease percentage of lean body mass and generalized muscle hypotrophy. These effects are related to the traditional remedy of this most cancers, which targets to block a super part of the circulating testosterone [7].

Lipolysis

In addition to growing lean mass, testosterone actively participates in lipolysis [8] (scientific name given to the lower in the period of adipocytes, and via extension to the shortage of fat). This impact is all the more important while the boom in testosterone is added approximately with the useful useful resource of sports activities interest - we are capable of see this in the next bankruptcy.

In addition, due to the truth that every adipocyte concentrates a huge quantity of estrogen, the lipolytic approach constitutes a form of virtuous circle: greater testosterone, a bargain much much less fat; tons a whole lot much less fat, more testosterone.

Libido, erectile feature and fertility

Notable high fine effects of testosterone on libido have been positioned in severa research. It might in all likelihood growth preference, fantasize's capability, similarly to the frequency of masturbation and sexual sex [9]. In addition, it might allow higher synthesis of nitric oxide, a molecule chargeable for the vasodilation of blood vessels: this effect must result in greater and longer erections. It changed into as a result observed that guys suffering from testosterone deficiency did no longer respond to Viagra, or handiest if it modified into followed with the useful useful resource of hormonal supplementation.

In addition, the worldwide lower in testosterone is going with a decrease in fertility. These markers are related: someone with a immoderate testosterone diploma may also moreover have a miles better chance of procreating than a negative man, despite the fact that the latter is supplementing himself.

Bone fitness

Testosterone facilitates bone health thru two mechanisms. The first is arguably the maximum counterintuitive, and consequences from the conversion of testosterone into estrogen - it sincerely is aromatization. Estrogen is crucial right right here, as it prevents all varieties of fractures and contamination [10]. The 2d, more traditional mechanism uses DHT, a herbal derivative of testosterone that reasons a massive growth in osteoblasts, those bone cells responsible for bone mineralization.

Again, research have decided that testosterone-horrible men are much more likely to interrupt any form of bone, and enjoy approximately two to 3 greater sprains than wholesome patients [11]. And if hormone opportunity treatment effects in an prolonged bone mineral density, it hasn't set up to lessen the risk of fracture in deficient subjects.

Mood

Testosterone improves mood and fights depression correctly: for instance, hormonal supplementation has been mounted to make poor men extra pleased and stimulated [12]. However, the motives for this correlation aren't however completely understood thru the studies community, and research are sometimes inconsistent and paradoxical.

We consequently preserve on with the primary statement, especially that testosterone efficaciously fights despair, although the results can be choppy depending on the profile.

Cognition

There are many androgenic receptors within the mind, which lets in testosterone to behave immediately on thoughts potential. Studies have verified that older guys with excessive testosterone score better on exams of memorization, visible-spatial instance, and language abilties than those inner or underneath the norm [13]. Conversely, ladies and men with a loss of testosterone are more likely to increase neurodegenerative illnesses, specifically Alzheimer's [14] and Parkinson's [15].

Diabetes and metabolic syndrome

Most guys with diabetes have low testosterone levels, and supplementation allows decorate blood sugar and pancreatic insulin reaction. Likewise, the better the testosterone degree in a subject, the decrease the risk of growing type 2 diabetes [16].

The equal goes for the metabolic syndrome, characterised by way of manner of fatty liver, extra ldl ldl cholesterol, and too much visceral fat: normal, a testosterone deficiency is associated with those three standards, at the same time as a excessive charge prevents their look. This high-quality motion is right away related to the lower in blood markers of infection: C-reactive protein, glycemia, ldl cholesterol and sedimentation rate [17].

Autoimmune ailments

On not unusual, ladies are twice as affected as guys with the aid of manner of autoimmune sicknesses. This is because of hormonal versions and the protection afforded through testosterone. By lowering infection and preventing overactivation of the immune system, its supplementation prevents the improvement of immoderate types of multiple sclerosis, ankylosing polyarthritis [18], lupus and Hashimoto's thyroiditis. And as testosterone levels decline with age, the danger of contracting an autoimmune disease will growth.

Other outcomes

Testosterone additionally decreases the hazard of contracting HIV [19], increases hairiness, self-self assurance, electricity, recognition ... To tell the truth, it'd take too prolonged to listing and broaden all of the beneficial outcomes of T!

These records talk for themselves: testosterone deficiency is undesirable, and should be prevented the least bit prices. Yet data advocate the opposite. Since the 1960s, Western guys have expert a non-forestall drop of their testosterone degrees - the fault of many elements that want to be developed within a 2d celebration.

Chapter 14: The western manner of life, the proper perpetrator

Screens, lack of sleep and exposure to waves

File to be lower again urgently, on line invoice manage, series no longer to be left out, YouTube video to be seen ... There isn't any scarcity of opportunities to examine over the monitors and postpone bedtime. Blame it on too entire a life, too demanding a project, too heavy obligations.

If the frame can adapt for some time at a staggered tempo, the element consequences aren't lengthy in being felt rapid. Fatigue, critical to irritability and tension in its wake, seems first; This effects in favored apathy, loss of cognizance, exacerbated ache, and, of course ... A decrease in testosterone.

Scientific research are unanimous in this assignment rely variety. In absolutely one among them, a cohort of young men turned into pressured to sleep only 5 hours a night time for in line with week. Result: on not unusual, there was a ten to 15% decrease of their testosterone diploma [20]. We will consequently ensure to sleep as a minimum 7 hours consistent with night, or extra if viable. If you're prone to insomnia, natural components will will let you get to sleep - and don't worry, daylight hours naps effectively make up for a awful night time time.

Furthermore, publicity to video show units is carefully associated with electromagnetic waves' publicity. Thus, it's been established that using the cell phone reduces the testosterone level and the motility of the spermatozoa, the fault of the waves emitted through it [21]. The equal conclusions had been stated for wi-fi waves [22].

So what to do? It is proper that it's far tough - if now not almost not viable - to break out the consequences of electromagnetic waves, besides you want to live in seclusion in a white place. The best solution is to show your self as little as feasible: you may placed your telephone in aircraft mode at the same time as now not in use, you may float your bed far from the internet box, you may hook up with Ethernet in choice to wi-fi, you'll keep away from the usage of too much 4G / 5G ...

By slumbering better and thru exposing yourself less to shows and waves, you improve a struggling testosterone degree: the results are usually quite speedy, and can be determined after a few weeks of alternate. And if that is however insufficient, it is a terrific begin.

The significance of exercising and frame fats percent

The lack of exercise is the alternative most vital trouble because of a Western way of life. Between artwork, children and amusement, we do no longer do not forget exercising often. However, exercise has many advantages: progressed cardiovascular health, prevention of diabetes, maintenance of bones ... And, you guessed it, expanded testosterone degrees.

This is particularly the case with strength schooling and HIIT - High-Intensity Interval Training. This technique includes severe physical training of spherical 30 seconds (cycling, strolling, rowing, and many others.) observed thru a better or equal lively restoration time. While cardio education will boom DHT by myself [23], HIIT additionally improves unfastened testosterone stages [24].

The blessings of bodily workout do now not prevent there: through burning power over the long term, the body receives rid of superfluous fat cells. In addition to storing fat, those cells are actual estrogen reservoirs, that is why overweight men normally have a propensity to have decrease testosterone ranges [25]. It is vital to undergo in thoughts that testosterone cannot flow freely inside the presence of an excessive amount of estrogen.

A HIIT exercise software program should therefore be set up. A strong basis might be to carry out 3 thirty-minute exercising physical games in step with week, that specialize in powerful recreation - the elliptical and rowing tool artwork high-quality.

Swimming is not endorsed, because of the reality at the same time as this interest promotes weight loss, the chemical compounds applied in swimming pool water motive a drop in testosterone [26]. Also be careful now not to exceed your limits: overtraining can also cause hormonal issues [27].

Here is a endorsed novice schooling plan:

Monday: 20-minutes HIIT (rower)

Tuesday: Rest

Wednesday: Rest

Thursday: 20 mins HIIT (on foot)

Friday: Rest

Saturday: 25 minutes HIIT (biking)

Sunday: Rest

When you'll be more professional, you may increase the time and trouble of your exercising sporting events.

A developing publicity to endocrine disruptors

Endocrine disruptors are anywhere. Literally. Tap water, food, hygiene and cleaning products ... All are infected through way of way of these molecules with hormone-mimetic houses. By changing testosterone, they disrupt the hormonal stability and hold many pathologies.

It is probably now not viable to need to take away them virtually, however there are many steps that can be taken to restriction their presence. Here is a list of products that include a massive quantity of endocrine disruptors and the best techniques to get rid of them.

Hygiene and maintenance products

Hygiene merchandise are the main supply of endocrine disruptors. The substances that compose them are frequently very numerous, and maximum of them come from laboratories or chemical industries. Paraben, for example, is found in maximum mass market shampoos. Studies have shown that it extensively decreases testosterone stages in healthful topics [28]. The identical goes for make-up, beauty products, cleaning soap, dishwashing liquid ... [29]

The handiest viable answer is avoidance: pick out out merchandise with few natural materials, try not to clean your hair each day, stay away from perfumes and shaving foam, surrender your deodorant to spray, keep away from fluoride toothpaste, and so on. In brief, keep as few volatile products as possible.

Teflon pans

It may also additionally moreover sound extraordinary, however Teflon (the call given to polytetrafluoroethylene) acts as a powerful endocrine disruptor. Some research have stated its functionality to lower testosterone; others have even validated that the use of

Teflon pans introduced approximately a lower in penis length [30]. This is partly because of a immoderate cooking temperature, so one can boom the hormone-mimetic results of Teflon tenfold. We will consequently use ceramic or stainless-steel stoves, extra steady for hormonal health.

Plastic

The big perpetrator of endocrine disruption. If this reputation sticks to its pores and pores and pores and skin, it's miles because of the fact studies have verified the toxicity of bisphenol A, determined in massive portions in plastic [31]. A sizeable scientific consensus having usual spherical this task, its estrogenic homes are actually properly installation.

So what can be done to keep away from plastic, and most importantly, heated plastic? Prefer glass tupperware; keep away from the intake of canned food; drink filtered or glass water; pick out out out stainless-steel cutlery; avoid all plastic bottles.

Bottled and faucet water

Water is likewise a ability trouble. Bottled water, first of all, because of the truth it's miles stored in plastic - as we have were given visible formerly. Tap water, then, because of the fact it's far polluted through the usage of way of the stays of drugs and abortion pills. The research community has lengthy struggled to denounce the strong presence of endocrine disruptors in faucet water, and masses of studies have corroborated their claims [32].

It is therefore essential to reveal to glass bottles, or to install a water filtration tool. In this regard, be cautious in no manner to move away a plastic water bottle within the sun, the warmth notably potentiating the consequences of endocrine disruptors.

Pesticides

Present in large quantities in conventional food, insecticides regularly cause excessive hormonal disturbances. Erectile disorder, muscle losing, gynecomastia, growth retardation ... The results are effective and severa [33].

Faced with this scourge, measures can be taken: consumption of food from natural or close by agriculture, home made vegetable garden, in depth cleansing with water... The harmfulness of insecticides need to now not be omitted. For records, the food most affected are complete grains (wheat, barley, oats), culmination and veggies (mainly berries, tomatoes and potatoes) and legumes.

Certain tablets

It isn't always unusual for a drug, even to be had without a prescription, to include many endocrine disruptors. This is especially the case with anti inflammatory capsules (ibuprofen, aspirin, cortisone) and proton pump inhibitors (PPIs) [34]. It is also frequently determined in clinical gadget: catheters, syringes, blood luggage ...

The pointers are easy: in case your clinical health practitioner has prescribed treatment to you, then take it. We cannot threat questionning a clinical prescription. However, be aware about the aspect results, and popularity on the relaxation of this manual.

Phytoestrogens

Mainly determined in soybeans and extremely good flora, along aspect lentils, beans or flax, phytoestrogens, thru binding to circulating testosterone, an motion similar to that of estrogen [35]. Their absorption isn't always new, however is extra critical than in the past due to cutting-edge cooking strategies, which generates indigestible and stored estrogenic plant.

In order to avoid phytoestrogens as an entire lot as viable, it is going to be vital to ferment legumes, soybeans and high quality plants; unique meals will virtually be excluded (see the subsequent monetary disaster on meals).

Finasteride and its derivatives

Used to address benign prostatic hyperplasia and hair loss, finasteride motives marked erectile illness and occasional testosterone [36]. This movement is because of the capability of finasteride to dam 5-alpha reductase, an enzyme chargeable for changing testosterone into DHT: its inhibition promotes an increase in estrogen stages, and consequently, in flip, a marked feminization.

Finasteride ought to in no way be discontinued when you have a prostate circumstance, but the chance / benefit balance seems to be terrible with baldness.

Industrial exposition

Products applied in chemical, metallurgical, agro-meals and automobile flora consist of the most risky endocrinian disruptors. Many employees are exposed to it, ultimately growing excessive ailments: most cancers, pneumonia, leukemia, and so on. Diseases which, of direction, are located via a drop in testosterone [37].

Note that residents living close to factories are also at risk. Of path, it's miles difficult to trade jobs or relocate, however being aware about the dangers is once more a need.

These few hints, coupled with the ones given above, can drastically change the life of individuals who take a look at them. Usually, a upward push in testosterone is visible most effective numerous weeks after they are set up vicinity. Are they sufficient? Perhaps. But, beyond its interest of pesticides, the diet regime want to moreover be adjusted with precision.

Chapter 15: Diet one zero one

Macronutrients, micronutrients and energy

Food is the opportunity crucial foundation for hormonal optimization. Many parameters can be optimized thru this bias, and some guys have an hobby in changing their consuming behavior.

Energy and blood sugar

The calorie is an electricity rate permitting the body to perform its important abilities. The hormonal gadget is mainly sensitive to caloric intake, and desires energy to characteristic efficaciously. For example, studies have linked finest calorie intake to prolonged testosterone levels. Conversely, a country of undernutrition is probably dangerous [38]. So ensure you consume enough and don't get hungry too frequently.

Be cautious, but, not to move overboard: a giant rise in blood sugar degrees, related to too much calorie consumption, could possibly will be predisposed to decrease testosterone tiers [39]. Moderation is the critical thing.

It is estimated that an individual female needs 1,800 power in step with day; an individual man, 2100. Of path, the ones values are not constant, and range in line with the bodily interest practiced, the morphology, the dominion of fitness... Many online tool will will can help you precisely recognize your desires day by day.

Carbohydrate, protein and fats: the 3 vital macronutrients

A calorie is not the whole lot: it originates from considered one of three macronutrients - carbohydrate, protein and fat.

1g of carbohydrate = 4kcal

1g of protein = 4kcal

1g of fats = 9kcal

These macronutrients also are crucial for the frame, which capabilities poorly within the event of a deficiency. The same goes for the hormonal tool: the latter desires a ordinary supply of carbohydrates, proteins and fats.

Numerous studies highlight the blessings of a weight loss plan rich in lipids [40]: by enhancing the extent of HDL ldl cholesterol, fats participate in a excellent boom in testosterone, which requires ldl ldl ldl cholesterol to be synthesized by using the business enterprise. This is especially the case of saturated fat, located in butter, chocolate or eggs; the information are a whole lot less smooth about mono and polyunsaturated fats.

As mentioned before, proteins and carbohydrates ought to not be located apart each: by way of using taking element in muscle increase and reducing blood cortisol levels, they decorate testosterone degrees [41]. A balance among these 3 macronutrients must consequently be determined, and that is why it's miles vital to diversify your eating regimen - a weight loss plan that could not be entire with out a enough consumption of nutrients and minerals.

Micronutrients

Vitamins and minerals, additionally known as micronutrients, participate in hormonal stability with the useful resource of supplying the frame with essential factors. Here is a listing of the maximum exciting micronutrients for the synthesis of testosterone:

Zinc [42]: seafood, organ meats, legumes, complete grains and nuts. Magnesium [43]: chocolate, nuts, buckwheat, nutritional yeast and peanuts.

Selenium [44]: Brazil nuts, fish, seafood and offal.

Calcium [45]: dairy products, almonds, sardine bones and positive mineral waters (Hépar, Courmayeur, Contrex, Quézac).

Iodine [46]: fish, seafood and seaweed. Also essential for the synthesis of thyroid hormones.

Vitamin E [47]: almonds, sunflower seeds, avocado, olive oil and wheat germ oil.

B nutrients [48]: animal merchandise, dietary yeast, whole grains and nuts.

Vitamin C [49]: cease result and greens, such as kiwi, orange, strawberries, raspberries and peppers.

Vitamin K [50]: animal offal (K2), leafy veggies, fermented soybeans and natto (K1, precursor of K2).

If nutrients and mineral supplementation is feasible (see subsequent financial disaster), it might be fantastic to achieve a super dietary intake via meals.

Foods to keep away from

Before going any further and recommending the extremely good meals to increase your testosterone tiers, you want to first take into account which of them can be harmful. In view of present day-day conduct, it isn't surprising that they may be numerous - so many that it might be no longer feasible to rely all of them. Here is already an in depth listing of those which you have to exclude from your diet.

Dairy products

Often praised for his or her calcium content cloth, dairy merchandise are, for the maximum issue, awful for testosterone. There are truely many hormones there, together with the well-known estrogen - recollect that milk and its derivatives are first of all meant for feeding more youthful calves.

It isn't always surprising to be aware that these massive quantities of hormones, effortlessly assimilated with the aid of the frame, are at the start of a hormonal imbalance. One have a observe concluded that milk consumption induced a lower in testosterone in a cohort of boys [51] - and this impact is stronger the better the milk product is fatty, the hormones being determined in fat .

So, what to pick out out to satisfy your calcium desires? There are masses of answers. Calcium water, almonds, enriched vegetable milks, sardine bones ... It is higher to show to those alternatives than to preserve to eat dairy merchandise, specifically on the identical time as we understand that they'll be likely to result in exceptional health problems.

Processed meat

The intake of processed meats often leads to a large decrease in testosterone, because of the presence of nitrites, endocrine disruptors and hormonal residues [52]. In younger guys, the consumption of processed meats because of this ends in impaired motility and sperm rely [53].

It will therefore be crucial to drop processed meat and turn to unprocessed one or, failing that, devour portions from natural farming.

Soybeans

Renowned for its feminizing movement, soy induces an boom in estrogen ranges - specifically if it's miles of business basis. Not all studies agree on whether this estrogenic impact simply consequences in a drop in testosterone, but in most instances that is what takes location [54].

We will consequently avoid ingesting soy in all its industrial organisation paperwork: vegetable milk, tofu, yogurt, cream ... We will choose out to expose to standard alternatives, together with natto: fermented soybeans, better digested and containing little estrogen, is a lot heaps a good deal much less of a trouble.

Sugar

Sugar is also to be banned. Raising glycemia disproportionately, its ordinary intake lowers testosterone. For example, a take a look at placed a drastic drop in testosterone in men who drank a sugary drink [55]. If alternatives exist - stevia, mountain honey, cinnamon, and masses of others. - the extremely good is probably to step by step do away with the sweet taste. Beware of processed merchandise, which incorporates sauces, sandwich bread or dry cakes, which continuously encompass a extra or lesser percentage of sugar.

Flax seeds

Recent research have highlighted the estrogenic outcomes of consuming flax seeds: given to guys with prostate maximum cancers, they reason a huge lower in testosterone [56]. This is due to their richness in lignans, polyphenols appearing as endocrine disruptors [57]. It would therefore make experience to save you consuming flax seeds, or as a minimum lessen it - because of the reality powerful effects on cardiovascular fitness have notwithstanding the truth that been confirmed.

Trans fatty acids

If, as visible above, the consumption of lipids promotes an increase in testosterone degrees, this is not the case with trans fatty acids. On the opposite: located in fried food, commercial enterprise food (desserts, burgers, candies, snacks) and dehydrated soups, they may be the reason of cardiovascular disease, diabetes, maximum cancers and, obviously, hormonal imbalances [58] . In order to keep actual T stages, care want to be taken to keep away from fried food and processed products as a good deal as viable. Buy raw!

Alcohol

Bad information for enthusiasts of wine, beer, cider and distinctive spirits: alcohol consumption is terrible for testosterone. Researchers have highlighted the estrogenic effects of ethanol, which is likewise accountable for an boom in cortisol [59]. This movement might be dose-based totally, and could range ordinary with the awesome of the alcohol ingested.

In all cases, moderation is wanted, because of the truth, in addition to reducing testosterone, alcohol promotes many illnesses - cirrhosis, maximum cancers, excessive blood pressure, coronary coronary coronary heart rhythm issues ... In precept, the identical goes for cigarettes (its results on testosterone could probable also be more harmful).

Gluten-primarily based completely components

Gluten-free diets are all of the rage? So lots the higher. Gluten is thought to boom prolactin levels to an abnormally excessive degree [60]. The trouble is that prolactin is a hormone concerned within the gadget of lactation and discount of sexual desire, on the identical time inhibiting the production of testosterone.

Foods containing gluten (in reality, specifically the ones made from wheat, spelled, rye, oats and barley) have to be prevented. Exit then breads, cakes, pastries and pastries.

Fortunately for foodies, gluten-unfastened flour-primarily based absolutely options exist, and in the meanwhile are to be had in any hypermarket.

Mint

Its sensitive taste does now not permit mint to break out this list: participating inside the synthesis of estrogen, it reasons a marked decrease in testosterone tiers and sperm viability [61]. Chewing gum, teas, sweets, lozenges, salads: avoid all arrangements that contain it.

Chapter 16: Polyunsaturated vegetable oils

Polyunsaturated vegetable oils, with out trouble used for cooking and seasoning, reason a drop in testosterone. In any case, this is the quit result of numerous clinical studies [62]. Their immoderate omega 6 content and the trans fatty acids that they increase in some unspecified time in the future of cooking assist create a seasoned-inflammatory environment, a vector of hormonal imbalances [63]. Sunflower, soy, corn, sesame, rapeseed and peanut oils need to consequently be prevented.

Prefer saturated and monounsaturated oils, which encompass coconut oil, olive oil, macadamia oil or avocado oil: greater stable at some point of cooking and bad in omega 6, they do not gift any unique threat and can be consumed at will.

Licorice

Rather similar to mint, licorice moreover motives a drop in testosterone - the fault of its estrogenic motion and its excessive content material cloth of effective polyphenols [64]. We will consequently ban it outright from our weight loss plan. Fortunately, there are generally few not unusual sources of licorice, besides in chocolates, natural teas, and a few organized merchandise. Therefore, be aware about the list of factors.

Sodas

Several research have highlighted the hyperlink amongst ordinary intake of sodas and a drop in testosterone [65]. This is specifically because of the immoderate sugar content of those liquids: causing a disproportionate spike in blood sugar, they disrupt the hormonal reputation and growth the chance of overweight and weight problems. It's better to drink unsweetened beverages, which includes lemon sparkling water or vegetable milks.

Foods too immoderate in fiber

All health specialists agree that fibers have an vital anti-inflammatory movement, and enhance many blood parameters, which includes blood stress, blood sugar and protein-C stages. However, whilst consumed in too large portions, they lower testosterone tiers [66]. Blame it on their compounds, which, by binding to androgenic hormones, save you testosterone from circulating freely.

It is consequently encouraged now not to devour too many fibrous food inside the equal meal. Mixtures of legumes (chickpeas, lentils, beans) and complete grains must consequently be averted, and the equal goes for great culmination and veggies (artichokes, peas, pears).

Foods to preference

After getting a stable rundown of what food are awful for testosterone, right right here's the listing of those to eat. Whether they are of animal or plant foundation, they have useful homes for hormonal stability and can be fed on without risk.

Eggs

Eggs are an extraordinary supply of protein, saturated fat, nutrition A, and ldl cholesterol [67]. Chosen natural, they includes omega 3, which sell the protection of suitable cardiovascular health. Egg's dietary richness contributes to the growth in testosterone [68] and makes it an great buddy of preference inner a balanced diet plan.

As said above, it is higher to shop for eggs from organic farming or, failing that, from a fowl raised in the outdoor: containing extra nutrients, they're additionally plenty less problem to antibiotic residues.

Olive oil

Rich in monounsaturated fatty acids and nutrition E, olive oil has anti-oxidant houses which make contributions to the synthesis of testosterone and to the health of the testes [69]. You can upload it anywhere (salads, sauces, seasoning), such as at the same time as cooking. Organic olive oil is the best, as business oil regularly comes from an unreliable aggregate that originated in Asia.

Almonds

Almonds, particularly rich in nutrients E, calcium and magnesium, are chargeable for higher fertility and a big growth in testosterone [70]. Helping even in times of erectile ailment manner to their nitric oxide content material, they may be determined in uncooked shape, mash, flour and shavings. Again, determine upon herbal almonds.

Dark chocolate

Scientific studies have prolonged tested the masculinizing capacity of chocolate [71]. Considered as an aphrodisiac, chocolate is wealthy in saturated fatty acids, magnesium and theobromine, a compound with an antidepressant effect. The better the cocoa content material fabric, the extra the motion of the chocolate: choose bars 75% or greater, or possibly, if you could, cocoa beans - you could find out them in specialized stores.

Offal

Liver, kidneys, thoughts, shank, tab ... The desire of offal is huge. Good records: rich in vitamins A, B and K2 and containing crucial minerals, all take part successfully within the synthesis of testosterone [72]. Be cautious, but, to eat elements from herbal farming, because of the reality there are often pollutants and antibiotic residues.

Oysters

Renowned for their aphrodisiac houses, oysters pay hobby an first-rate amount of zinc. Studies have confirmed their capability to seriously growth testosterone stages, particularly in young guys [73]. So do no longer definitely save them for unique sports - your fitness and your fishmonger will thanks.

Beef

Also containing large portions of zinc, pork is rich in nutrients and essential amino acids. Consumed fats, it permits rebalance a marked testosterone deficit [74]. Organically farmed cuts are, once more, first rate to manufacturing unit-farmed red meat, ate up tablets and hormones.

Garlic

In addition to containing many anti-oxidants and exerting an anti-inflammatory movement, garlic stimulates the manufacturing of testosterone [75]. This impact is because of its content cloth cloth of allicin, an organosulfur compound acting at the reproductive machine, immunity, cognition and digestion [76]. Consumed undeniable, as a seasoning or in a salad, garlic is bendy and much less costly.

Ginger

The most crucial bio-energetic problem of ginger, 6-gingerol, is concept to be the motive of an growth in testosterone and nitric oxide degrees, consistent with the medical community [77]. Ideal for impotence, muscular hypotrophy and fatigue, ginger may be eaten in salads or as a seasoning.

Sardines

Sardines consist of omega 3, iodine, bones (a source of calcium) and excessive fine protein [78]. Low in heavy metals, their normal intake (approximately 2 to three instances in step with week) is usually recommended so that you can reach the iodine quota, essential for the producing of testosterone [79]. Tip: a great manner to multiply its masculinizing impact, taste them with olive oil.

Crucifers

Crucifers have very strong anti-estrogenic houses. Thus, in topics who've consumed cabbage, there can be an expanded urinary excretion of estrogen, in fact contributing to an increase in testosterone [80]. Cabbage, then, however furthermore radishes, beets, broccoli, turnips, watercress ... There are lots of alternatives.

Be careful not to consume an excessive amount of frequently: ingested in huge quantities, crucifers save you the absorption of iodine by means of using the body [81].

Onions

According to a systematic meta-have a take a look at, the intake of onion should cause a main surge in testosterone, and may make a contribution to sexual well-being, fertility as well as testicular fitness - its quercetin content cloth is probably the principle motive [82]. We will consequently take care to frequently add onions to our number one dishes, so long as they will be now not heated to too excessive a temperature, the cooking changing their nutritional charge.

Buckwheat

Arguably one of the most thrilling grains, buckwheat carries magnesium, zinc and copper in massive amounts [83]. Its everyday consumption permits preserve a excessive testosterone stage. Buckwheat is normally located in natural shops inside the shape of flakes, flakes or complete grains.

Gluten free oats

Praised for its excessive zinc content material material, oats take part inside the stimulation of testosterone with the aid of using acting right away at the manufacturing of nitric oxide [84]. It can be eaten as an entire cereal, bread, dry cake, or perhaps vegetable milk. Be careful to pick out out out it gluten unfastened - endure in thoughts the preceding element regarding gluten and prolactin upward thrust.

Brazil nuts

Brazil nuts are a very exciting source of selenium; in reality, excellent one is sufficient to fulfill the each day goals (be cautious for overdose) [85]. Involved in thyroid and hormonal fitness, their format and cheaper fee cause them to a top rate snack.

Honey

By attenuating cellular oxidation and inhibiting the aromatization machine, honey not without delay will growth the extent of testosterone [86]. For records, honey moreover has a amazing effect on cardiovascular fitness and stops the dangers of diabetes and excessive blood stress. Prefer natural and dark honeys, an lousy lot less rich in sugar.

Grapes

Naturally observed in grapes, trans-Resveratrol, in addition to stopping metabolic syndrome, is without delay involved inside the manufacturing of testosterone and various androgens [87]. Red grapes additionally seem like extra worried (as traditional, we can pick out them if feasible of natural beginning).

Pomegrenates

Native to Central Asia, pomegranate is a fruit ate up for thousands of years with the beneficial aid of the human beings of Jordan. Praised for its aphrodisiac virtues, its juice growth testosterone tiers, fight depression, reduce blood stress and the risk of cardiovascular sickness [88]. Whole or within the form of juice, pomegranate appears to be best as part of a hormonal rebalancing.

Mushrooms

Mushrooms, and further particularly button mushrooms, seem to efficiently inhibit aromatase interest, thereby lowering estrogen levels [89]. Due to its isoflavone content cloth, this effect is reduced on the identical time as the mushrooms are cooked, and willing while they're grilled.

Watermelon

Watermelon consists of immoderate quantities of flavonoids and arginine[90], and besides having anti-oxidant houses, it improves the satisfactory of erections and could boom testosterone level.

Chapter 17: Habits evaluation

Useful nutritional dietary supplements

As their call shows, nutritional dietary supplements do no longer update a balanced weight loss program or a healthful lifestyle, however can be beneficial as a part of an already optimized manner of lifestyles. Here is a non-exhaustive choice of dietary supplements that sell testosterone manufacturing.

Vitamins and minerals: already mentioned in the preceding financial ruin, first-class vitamins and minerals can rebalance a testosterone deficiency. The most exciting are zinc, magnesium, copper, weight loss program A, weight loss program E, food plan K2 MK4, weight loss plan C, B vitamins, calcium and iodine (most effective in case you are terrible).

Fenugreek: 1000-12 months-antique medicinal plant, fenugreek, constant with severa research [91], will increase the testosterone stage of male contributors.

Ashwagandha: Also known as Indian ginseng, ashwagandha participates within the synthesis of testosterone [92].

Creatine: Creatine not immediately will increase testosterone degrees through selling its conversion into DHT and inhibiting the aromatization system [93].

Boron: truly determined in effective stop end result, veggies and nuts (eg mushrooms, broccoli, potatoes, hazelnuts), boron is a hint element lowering estrogen stages while developing the ones of unfastened testosterone [94]. Supplementation is specially indicated if there can be a dietary deficiency.

Ginseng: A clinical meta-look at concluded that ginseng stimulates testosterone manufacturing, protects sperm from capacity oxidative harm, and improves male fertility [95].

Luteolin: Also called luteolol, luteolin is a flavonoid that promotes the manufacturing of sperm and testosterone [96]. Found in celery, thyme and dandelion, a complement is frequently higher dosed and extra powerful.

Mucuna: Mucuna, or bagpipe, inhibits cortisol levels, allows in testosterone synthesis, and increases sperm matter wide variety and motility in terrible men [97].

Yohimbine: An alkaloid derived from the bark of yohimbe, a West African tree, yohimbine efficaciously fights erectile sickness and pretty will growth testosterone levels [98].

Chrysin: Chrysin, a flavonoid absolutely located in blue passionflower, allows preserve a healthy hormonal stability with the resource of in component blockading the conversion of testosterone to estrogen [99].

Omega 3: thanks to their anti inflammatory movement, omega protects spermatozoa from oxidative damage and restores low testosterone tiers [100]. Take them in case you do no longer eat - or a hint - oily fish.

Tongkat ali: a virulent disease plant nearby to Indonesia, Tongkat Ali induces an growth in testosterone and an improvement in inflammatory markers [101], allowing horrible guys to regain a normal splendid of existence.

Shilajit: extracted from rock and mineral and herbal remember range, shijalit can also need to drastically increase the volume of androgenic hormones and permit testosterone to flow into greater freely [102].

Burdock: a huge plant located anywhere in the global, burdock will growth sperm production, decreases prolactin, improves fertility and enables keep a excessive testosterone degree [103].

Techniques that without a doubt artwork

Beyond food plan, supplementation and an top of the road way of lifestyles, the adoption of severa techniques may be useful. The following listing has intentionally set apart techniques which can be more myth than reality; only those that have been set up via the scientific community continue to be.

Wear unfastened undies: a large American have a have a look at related to more than 650 contributors has hooked up that sporting free boxers promotes sperm production and improves fertility; conversely, tight undies became risky to testicular and hormonal characteristic [104]. This is because of the truth the testes want a pretty low temperature to feature successfully [105]. So avoid briefs, and alternatively placed on loose briefs and boxers.

Exposure to the sun: considering the truth that weight loss program D promotes the manufacturing of testosterone, everyday exposure to the sun might be to opposite a capacity hormonal imbalance [106]. Vitamin D dietary dietary supplements may be useful in wintry climate, however are not an opportunity desire to natural exposure. Be cautious no longer to extend the latter too long, as it's miles the main reason of pores and pores and skin maximum cancers [107]. Also keep away from traditional sunscreens, too wealthy in chemical materials, and prefer herbal alternatives.

Take bloodless showers: both praised and criticized, this technique may be powerful [108], furnished that the shower is neither too long nor too cold, in any other case the blood cortisol degree will boom. As noted in advance, the testes want a low temperature to correctly produce sperm, and cool water stimulates testosterone production domestically.

Perform severa units of squats: as we have seen, physical exercise is beneficial for hormonal fitness. This is in particular real on the subject of muscle education for the legs: numerous studies have really validated that appearing several units of squats substantially increases testosterone tiers [109]. Virtually performable everywhere, squats also can also be finished the use of extra weights.

Maintain an lively sex life: Several researchers have claimed that an energetic and eye-catching sex lifestyles promotes prolonged testosterone manufacturing and contributes to sperm viability [110], even in older guys.

Intermittent fasting: intermittent fasting consists of spacing out meals consumption through the usage of at least 12 hours, the traditional sample at the side of fasting approximately sixteen hours consistent with day (from eight p.M. To noon, for example). Studies have proven that, while practiced very well, intermittent fasting can modestly stimulate testosterone manufacturing [111]. Be cautious, but, now not to speedy for too prolonged, nor to below-nourish your self. As visible in the 2d financial wreck, a country of undernutrition significantly disrupts the hormonal stability of the organism. A fast lasting 12 to sixteen hours need to consequently be advanced.

Drink coffee often: in line with severa research, coffee reasons an boom in free testosterone and a decrease in estrogen levels [112]. Men who eat espresso often are for that reason possibly to have better testosterone degrees than non-drinkers [113]. Be cautious, however, not to overdo it: in too huge a amount, caffeine will boom cortisol and disrupts the hormonal balance. One cup in step with day is the encouraged dose.

Support a winning team: inside the lower back of this fascinating expression hides a truth this is just as lots: in step with the medical community, witnessing a victory for your preferred organization may notably growth testosterone ranges [114]. The turn side is that a defeat would possibly produce the alternative impact - specially a decline in androgens. So make certain of your bet.

Choose your films cautiously : From a whole have a take a look at, the researchers confirmed that individuals looking films categorised as competitive, erotic and athletic skilled a moderate rise in testosterone; conversely, folks who had watched suffered a sad hormonal decrease and were extra pressured [115].

Testosterone Replacement Therapy (TRT)

In some very particular instances, even the brilliant will inside the worldwide can fail to correct a testosterone deficiency. This setback highlights an underlying fitness hassle that should be treated with the assist of a scientific expert.

TRT, an desire to be considered as a final lodge

TRT, or Testosterone Replacement Therapy, is a specially famous exercising in Anglo-Saxon international places. It consists of restoring abnormally low hormonal degrees through often injecting synthetic testosterone [116].

In the usa, many guys use it as early as their fortieth 3 hundred and sixty five days, in spite of the truth that they do now not have a specific disability. This affords a large danger, because of the truth the deliver of exogenous testosterone disrupts the hypothalamic-pituitary thyroid axis and prevents the body from truely generating androgenic hormones; from time to time this effect is irreversible [117].

Obtainable great on medical prescription in most countries, TRT is indicated in the outstanding case wherein a ailment reasons a sufficiently marked decline of testosterone. If you watched that is the case, see your clinical medical doctor; the medical doctor will prescribe blood checks and, if vital, hormonal treatment. Otherwise, really undertake herbal and risk-unfastened techniques.